# ALLERGY FREE
## FAMILY FAVORITES

CHEF
BRIAN
HACKBARTH

Visit www.booksurge.com to order additional copies.

# Table of Contents

## Pork

## Pastas

## Vegetables

## Sides

## Soups

## Salads

# Forward

The goal of this book is for families to enjoy one delicious meal together, whether or not each family member has food allergies.  That is why not just some, but *every* recipe in this book is free of wheat, dairy, eggs, peanuts, tree nuts, fish, shellfish, sesame and soy.  For those without food allergies, this book will provide an extremely tasteful and healthy collection of recipes.  I hope you find the way I wrote each recipe easy to follow.  I tried to make them as simple as possible.  By listing the ingredients first in each recipe you already have your shopping list.  The preparation section of each recipe flows in the same order the ingredients are listed, which should help you to not miss any steps and make the recipes in the least amount of time.  Though no one in my family has food allergies, we eat these foods on a daily basis and I have found weight loss to be an extra benefit.  I hope you find these recipes as easy to make and delicious as my family and friends do.

# Disclaimer

If you have questions about whether or not you can eat the foods in this book, you should consult with your allergist or doctor.  I am neither of those.  I have no responsibility or liability for use of these recipes.  People using this cookbook must check the safety of all ingredients with an allergist or other doctor.

# About the Author

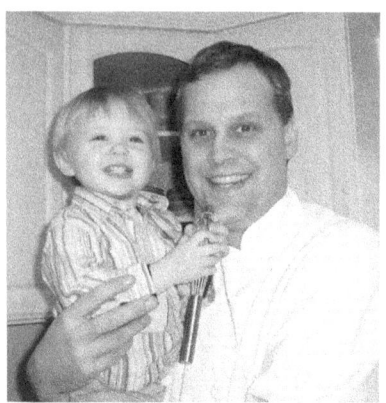

**Chef Brian Hackbarth**

I began working in the culinary field after discovering that my original career in marketing and sales was unfulfilling and my true passion was cooking. In 1998 I returned to college and earned a culinary degree with honors from Joliet Junior College. I honed my culinary skills at Elgin Country Club in Elgin, Illinois. At the club I created a daily appetizer, pasta and fish special and oversaw the preparation and presentation of meals for weddings and private parties. Following my time at the country club, I decided to start Relish The Night Personal Chef Services. As a personal chef I find that my love for food, creative menu planning skills and ability to work with people allow me to provide an outstanding service to my clients. I cook for upscale private cocktail and dinner parties, teach cooking classes and prepare weekly meals for families with busy lifestyles.

When a friend with food allergies alerted me to the problems families experience in preparing a healthy, non-allergenic meal, I decided to write this cookbook. As a stay at home dad I understand the time constraints in running a household and created this book to help ease the pressure these families face. The fact that many cook two meals each time the family eats is one of the main problems. My hope is to decrease the time spent deciding what to cook, shopping and preparing meals and increase the time the entire family spends enjoying their meals together.

# Acknowledgements

I would like to thank my wife Mary for her love, patience and understanding. Thanks also to my mom Suzanne for spending time with Brody as I developed and typed recipes. The time each of you spent testing and proofreading recipes helped immensely. Without your help I would have never gotten this accomplished. I also wanted to thank my son Brody who helped inspire me to write this cookbook. I love and appreciate all of you.

# Commonly Used Items

One of the ideas behind this book is to use the same items in a variety of recipes. That way if your pantry is stocked, you have multiple dinner options. This helps take the pressure off the meal provider by having foods available that the entire family can enjoy together.

# Equipment:

Baking sheet
Candy thermometer
Dutch oven
Large pot
Large sauté pan
Measuring cups
Measuring spoons
Meat thermometer
Oven thermometer
Ricer
Two-quart pan with lid
Whisk
Wire cooling rack
Zester

# Pantry Items:

Balsamic vinegar
Barbeque sauce
Bay leaves
Beef broth
Black pepper
Brown rice pasta
Canola oil
Chicken broth
Chili powder
Cornstarch
Cumin
Dijon mustard
Dried basil
Dried oregano
Dried French thyme
Extra virgin olive oil
Garlic powder
Kosher salt
Light brown sugar
Long grain white rice
Paprika
Rice wine vinegar
Sun-dried tomatoes
Vegetable oil
White wine vinegar

# Keys To Success In The Kitchen

1. Read the entire recipe before you begin.
2. Have all of your preparation done before you start to cook.
3. Have an oven thermometer inside your oven to check the accuracy of the desired cooking temperature.
4. Always pre-heat your oven for a minimum of 30 minutes.
5. Always pre-heat your grill for a minimum of 15 minutes with the lid closed.
6. When taking meats out of the oven or off the grill, let them "rest" 5-20 minutes wrapped with aluminum foil prior to serving or carving.
7. Take all meats out of the refrigerator and set them on the counter 15-30 minutes to come to room temperature prior to cooking.
8. Do not overcook foods.
9. Always taste foods prior to serving and adjust seasonings if needed.
10. Have Fun, Serve Great Food and Enjoy!

# Chapter 1 | **Spice Mixes**

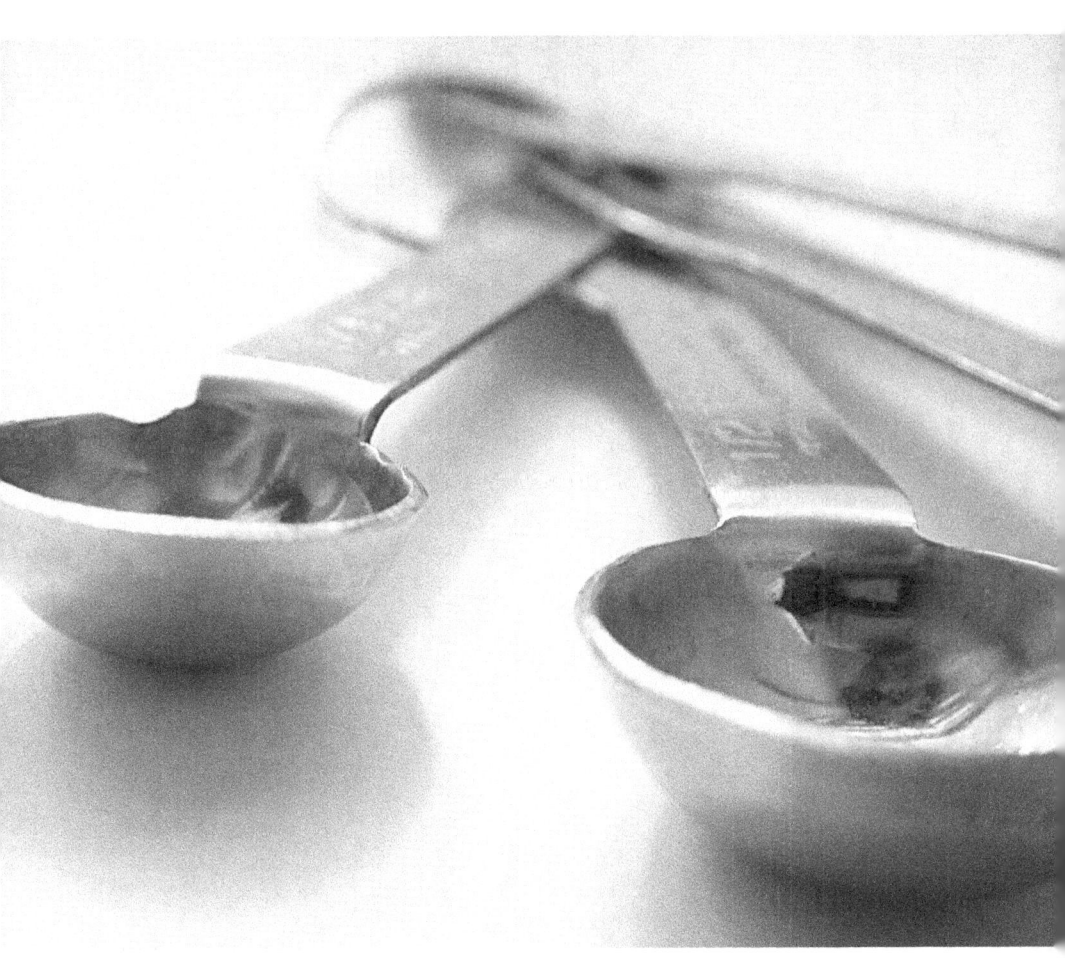

# SPG Mix

## Ingredients:

1. 1 cup kosher salt
2. 1 tablespoon freshly ground black pepper
3. 1 tablespoon garlic powder

## Preparation:

1. Combine all ingredients in an air tight container
2. Close container and shake to combine ingredients
3. Store in a cool dry place
4. Use to season all foods

# Mexican Spice Mix

## Ingredients:

1. 4 tablespoons kosher salt
2. 4 tablespoons paprika
3. 4 tablespoons chili powder
4. 2 tablespoons ground cumin
5. 2 tablespoons garlic powder
6. 1½ teaspoons freshly ground black pepper

## Preparation:

1. Combine all ingredients in an air tight container
2. Close container and shake to combine ingredients
3. Store in a cool dry place

# Chapter 2 | **Beef**

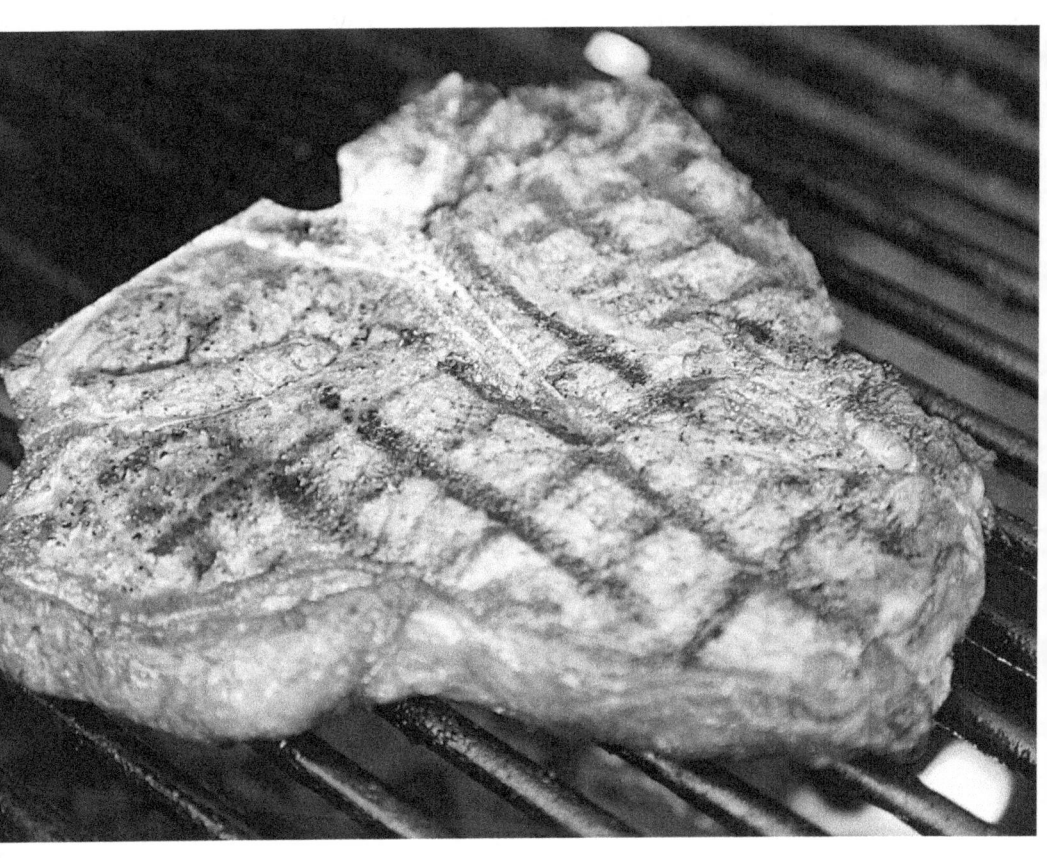

# Marinated Filet Mignon

## Ingredients:

1. 3 garlic cloves
2. 2 tablespoons packed fresh thyme
3. 2 tablespoons packed fresh tarragon
4. 2 tablespoons packed light brown sugar
5. 1½ tablespoons balsamic vinegar
6. 1 tablespoon paprika
7. ½ teaspoon fresh cracked black pepper
8. 1¼ teaspoon SPG mix (divided 1 teaspoon and ¼ teaspoon)
9. 2 tablespoons extra-virgin olive oil
10. 4 six-ounce filet mignons

## Preparation:

1. Puree garlic and put in a mixing bowl
2. Fine chop thyme and tarragon and add to bowl
3. Add brown sugar, balsamic vinegar, paprika, black pepper, 1 teaspoon SPG mix and olive oil to bowl and whisk together
4. Put steaks in a large resealable bag, add marinade and seal
5. Marinate in refrigerator 30 minutes to 2 hours
6. Take steaks out of refrigerator and set on counter 20 minutes prior to cooking
7. Pre-heat grill over a medium-high flame 15 minutes

## Cooking:

1. Remove steaks from marinade and put directly on grill
2. Season steaks with remaining ¼ teaspoon SPG mix
3. Grill steaks 4 minutes
4. Rotate steaks 90 degrees and grill 2 minutes
5. Flip steaks over and grill 3 minutes for medium-rare, 4 minutes for medium, 5 minutes for medium-well and 6 minutes for well done
6. Take steaks off grill, cover with aluminum foil and let rest 5 minutes
7. Serve and enjoy

# Flank Steak with Sweet Onions

## Ingredients:

1. 2 yellow onions
2. 1 garlic clove
3. 1¾ teaspoons SPG mix (divided ¾ teaspoon and 1 teaspoon)
4. ¾ teaspoon dried thyme (divided ½ teaspoon and ¼ teaspoon)
5. 3 tablespoons extra-virgin olive oil (divided 1 tablespoon and 2 tablespoons)
6. 1¼ pounds flank steak
7. ½ cup apricot jam

## Preparation:

1. Thinly slice onions and set aside
2. Puree garlic and put in a small bowl
3. Add ¾ teaspoon SPG mix, ½ teaspoon thyme and 1 tablespoon olive oil to garlic and mix together
4. Evenly rub mixture over top of steak and set aside
5. Pre-heat grill over a medium-high flame 15 minutes

**Cooking:**

1. Pre-heat a large sauté pan over a medium-high flame 2 minutes
2. Add remaining 2 tablespoons olive oil and heat 30 seconds
3. Add onions and sauté 5 minutes stirring occasionally
4. Add remaining 1 teaspoon SPG mix and ¼ teaspoon thyme and sauté 5 minutes stirring occasionally
5. Add apricot jam and stir to combine
6. Turn flame to low and hold onion mixture until needed to top steak
7. Grill steak 5 minutes
8. Flip steak over and grill 5 minutes
9. Remove steak from grill, cover with aluminum foil and let rest 5 minutes
10. Thinly slice steak against grain
11. Plate steak and top each portion with onion mixture
12. Serve and enjoy

# Beef Brisket

## Ingredients:

1. 1 yellow onion
2. 2 carrots
3. 3 garlic cloves
4. 1 tablespoon Mexican spice mix
5. 1 tablespoon SPG mix
6. 1 four-pound beef brisket
7. 2 tablespoons extra-virgin olive oil
8. 3 bay leaves
9. 1 cup beef broth
10. 1 cup water
11. 2 tablespoons ketchup

## Preparation:

1. Pre-heat oven to 350 degrees
2. Large dice onion and carrots and set aside
3. Peel garlic, smash cloves open and add to onions and carrots
4. Combine Mexican spice mix and SPG mix in a small bowl
5. Rub spices over entire brisket

## Cooking:

1. Pre-heat a Dutch oven over a high flame 1 minute
2. Add olive oil
3. Sear brisket fat side down 2 minutes
4. Flip brisket and sear 2 minutes
5. Add onions, carrots, garlic, bay leaves, beef broth, water and ketchup and bring to a boil
6. Cover with lid, put in oven and braise 3 hours (until fork tender)
7. Remove brisket from oven and let rest 15 minutes
8. Place brisket fat side down on cutting board
9. Thinly slice against grain
10. Serve and enjoy

# Barbecue Beef Brisket

## Ingredients:

1. 2 tablespoons Mexican spice mix
2. 1 four-pound beef brisket
3. 2 tablespoons extra-virgin olive oil
4. 1 cup tomato juice
5. 1 cup water
6. 2½ cups barbecue sauce (divided ½ cup and 2 cups)

## Preparation:

1. Pre-heat oven to 350 degrees
2. Evenly rub Mexican spice mix over entire brisket

**Cooking:**

1. Pre-heat a Dutch oven over a high flame 1 minute
2. Add olive oil
3. Sear brisket fat side down 2 minutes
4. Flip brisket and sear 2 minutes
5. Add tomato juice and water and bring to a boil
6. Pour ½ cup barbeque sauce over brisket
7. Cover with lid, put in oven and braise 3 hours (until fork tender)
8. Remove brisket from oven and let rest 15 minutes
9. In a small saucepan, warm remaining 2 cups barbeque sauce over a low flame
10. Place brisket fat side down on cutting board
11. Thinly slice against grain
12. Plate brisket topped with warmed barbeque sauce
13. Serve and enjoy

TIP: Brisket can easily be made ahead of lime. If so, refrigerate brisket whole after cooking and thinly slice prior to re-heating. To re-heat, top brisket with barbeque sauce and warm in a 300 degree oven.

# Beef Bourguignon

## Ingredients:

1. 1 small yellow onion
2. 12 ounces button mushrooms
3. 3 garlic cloves
4. 3 pounds chuck steak
5. 1½ teaspoons SPG mix (divided 1 teaspoon and ½ teaspoon)
6. 1 teaspoon dried French thyme
7. 3 bay leaves
8. 1 cup red wine
9. 2 tablespoons ketchup
10. 1 tablespoon balsamic vinegar
11. 4 cups beef broth
12. 6 tablespoons cornstarch
13. 4 tablespoons water
14. 1 tablespoon extra-virgin olive oil

## Preparation:

1. Small dice onion and put in a bowl
2. Quarter button mushrooms and add to bowl
3. Puree garlic and add to bowl
4. Trim fat off steak and cut into ¾ inch cubes
5. Season cubes of steak with 1 teaspoon SPG mix
6. Combine cornstarch and water, whisk together and set aside

## Cooking:

1. Pre-heat a large pot over a high flame 1 minute
2. Add olive oil and heat 30 seconds
3. Add steak and sear 2 minutes
4. Stir steak and sear remaining sides, about 2 minutes
5. Add onions, mushrooms and garlic, stir and sauté 4 minutes
6. Add remaining ½ teaspoon SPG mix, thyme, bay leaves, red wine, ketchup and balsamic vinegar
7. Bring to a boil and reduce 5 minutes
8. Add broth and bring to a boil
9. When it reaches a boil, turn flame to low and simmer 30 minutes
10. Whisk cornstarch and water into sauce
11. Bring to a boil and simmer 5 minutes
12. Take out bay leaves
13. Serve and enjoy

TIP: Great served over Mashed Yukon Gold Potatoes page 132

# Grilled New York Strip Steak

## Ingredients:

1. 4 eight-ounce New York strip steaks
2. 2 tablespoons packed light brown sugar
3. 1 tablespoon extra-virgin olive oil
4. ¾ teaspoon SPG mix (divided ½ teaspoon and ¼ teaspoon)
5. ¼ teaspoon dried French thyme

## Preparation:

1. Combine brown sugar, olive oil, ½ teaspoon SPG mix and thyme in a bowl and mix to form a paste
2. Evenly rub paste over one side of each steak and leave steaks on counter
3. Pre-heat grill over a medium-high flame 15 minutes

## Cooking:

1. Put steaks on grill paste side down
2. Season other side of steak with remaining ¼ teaspoon SPG mix and grill 4 minutes
3. Rotate steaks 90 degrees and grill 2 minutes
4. Flip steaks over and grill 3 minutes for medium-rare, 4 minutes for medium, 5 minutes for medium-well and 6 minutes for well done
5. Take steaks off grill, cover with aluminum foil and let rest 5 minutes
6. Serve and enjoy

TIP: Serve with Bacon, Onion and Mushroom Topping page 18

# Bacon, Onion and Mushroom Topping

## Ingredients:

1. 4 slices bacon
2. 1 tablespoon extra-virgin olive oil
3. 1 yellow onion
4. 8 ounces button mushrooms
5. 1 garlic clove
6. 1 teaspoon SPG mix

## Preparation:

1. Freeze bacon 10 minutes (this makes cutting very easy)
2. Dice onion and put in a bowl
3. Slice mushrooms and add to bowl
4. Puree garlic and set aside
5. Take bacon out of freezer, slice into ¼ inch wide strips and set aside

**Cooking:**

1. Pre-heat a large sauté pan over a medium-high flame 1 minute
2. Add bacon and sauté 1 minute
3. Add olive oil, onions and mushrooms and sauté 5 minutes stirring occasionally
4. Season with SPG mix, turn flame to medium and sauté 5 minutes stirring occasionally
5. Add garlic and sauté 2 minutes stirring occasionally
6. Serve and enjoy

# Hamburger

## Ingredients:

1. ¼ cup yellow onion
2. ¼ cup red pepper
3. ½ teaspoon garlic powder
4. 2 tablespoons barbeque sauce
5. 1 teaspoon SPG mix (divided ¾ teaspoon and ¼ teaspoon)
6. 1¼ pounds ground beef

## Preparation:

1. Small dice onion and put in a mixing bowl
2. Small dice pepper and add to bowl
3. Add garlic powder, barbeque sauce, ¾ teaspoon SPG mix and ground beef to bowl and mix together
4. Form 4 equal sized burgers and use your thumb to make an indentation in center of each burger (an indentation keeps burgers from plumping up in center)
5. Place burgers on a plate, wrap with plastic and refrigerate 15 minutes
6. Pre-heat grill over a medium-high flame 15 minutes
7. Remove burgers from refrigerator and season with remaining ¼ teaspoon SPG mix

## Cooking:

1. Grill burgers 5 minutes on each side, flipping only once
2. Remove burgers from grill
3. Serve and enjoy

TIP: Hamburgers can be broiled on high 5 minutes per side on a foil lined baking sheet

This burger is great topped with Bacon, Onion and Mushroom Topping page 18 or Grilled Onions page 22

# Grilled Onions

## Ingredients:

1. 2 large yellow onions
2. 1 tablespoon extra-virgin olive oil
3. ½ teaspoon SPG mix

## Preparation:

1. Slice ends off onions and peel away skins
2. Slice onions into ¼ inch thick discs
3. Drizzle each disc with olive oil and season with SPG mix
4. Pre-heat grill over a medium-high flame 15 minutes

## Cooking:

1. Grill onions 3 minutes on each side, flipping only once
2. Remove onions from grill
3. Serve and enjoy

TIP:  Great on top of Hamburger page 20

# Caramelized Onions

## Ingredients:

1. 2 large yellow onions
2. 3 tablespoons extra-virgin olive oil
3. ½ teaspoon SPG mix

## Preparation:

1. Thinly slice onions and set aside

**Cooking:**

1. Pre-heat a large sauté pan over a medium-high flame 2 minutes
2. Add olive oil and heat 30 seconds
3. Add onions and sauté 3 minutes without stirring or moving pan
4. Stir onions and sauté 5 minutes
5. Season with SPG mix, stir and sauté 5 minutes
6. Serve and enjoy

Great with grilled steak, chicken or burgers

# Steak Fajitas

## Ingredients:

1. 2 yellow onions
2. 1 red pepper
3. 1 green pepper
4. 2 jalapeño peppers
5. 2 garlic cloves
6. zest of 1 lime
7. 1 tablespoon packed light brown sugar
8. 2½ tablespoons Mexican spice mix (divided 1 tablespoon and 1½ tablespoons)
9. 3 tablespoons extra-virgin olive oil (divided 1½ tablespoons and 1½ tablespoons)
10. 1¼ pounds flank steak
11. ½ teaspoon freshly ground black pepper
12. 1 teaspoon fresh lime juice

## Preparation:

1. Thinly slice onions and set aside
2. Thinly slice red and green peppers and put in a bowl
3. Fine dice jalapeños and add to bowl
4. Puree garlic and set aside
5. Zest lime and put zest in a small bowl
6. Add brown sugar, 1 tablespoon Mexican spice mix and 1½ tablespoons olive oil to lime zest and mix to form a paste
7. Evenly rub paste over one side of steak and set steak aside
8. Grind black pepper and set aside
9. Pre-heat grill over a medium-high flame 15 minutes

## Cooking:

1. Pre-heat a large sauté pan over a medium-high flame 1 minute
2. Add remaining 1½ tablespoons olive oil
3. Add onions and sauté 4 minutes
4. Add peppers and sauté 4 minutes
5. Add garlic and remaining 1½ tablespoons Mexican spice mix and sauté 2 minutes
6. Add lime juice and hold vegetables over a low flame while steak cooks
7. Put steak on grill paste side down
8. Season other side of steak with black pepper and grill 5 minutes
9. Flip steak over and grill 5 minutes
10. Remove steak from grill and let rest 5 minutes
11. Thinly slice steak against grain and add to vegetables
12. Serve and enjoy

TIP: Fajitas are best with warmed brown rice tortillas and Guacamole page 149

# Beef Tacos

## Ingredients:

1. 1½ pounds ground beef
2. 1 red onion
3. 1 red pepper
4. 1 green pepper
5. 2 jalapeño peppers
6. 2 garlic cloves
7. 3 tablespoons Mexican spice mix
8. ½ cup packed fresh cilantro
9. 1 cup tomato juice
10. 1 tablespoon fresh lime juice

## Preparation:

1. Small dice onion and put in a bowl
2. Small dice red and green peppers and add to bowl
3. Fine dice jalapeños and add to bowl
4. Puree garlic and add to bowl
5. Fine chop cilantro and set aside

## Cooking:

1. Pre-heat a large sauté pan over a medium-high flame 1 minute
2. Add ground beef and sauté 5 minutes
3. Add onion, peppers, garlic and Mexican spice mix, stir and sauté 3 minutes
4. Add cilantro, tomato juice and lime juice
5. Bring to a boil and simmer 5 minutes
6. Serve and enjoy

TIP: I like with warmed soft shell corn tortillas and Pico De Gallo page 148

# Chapter 3 | Chicken

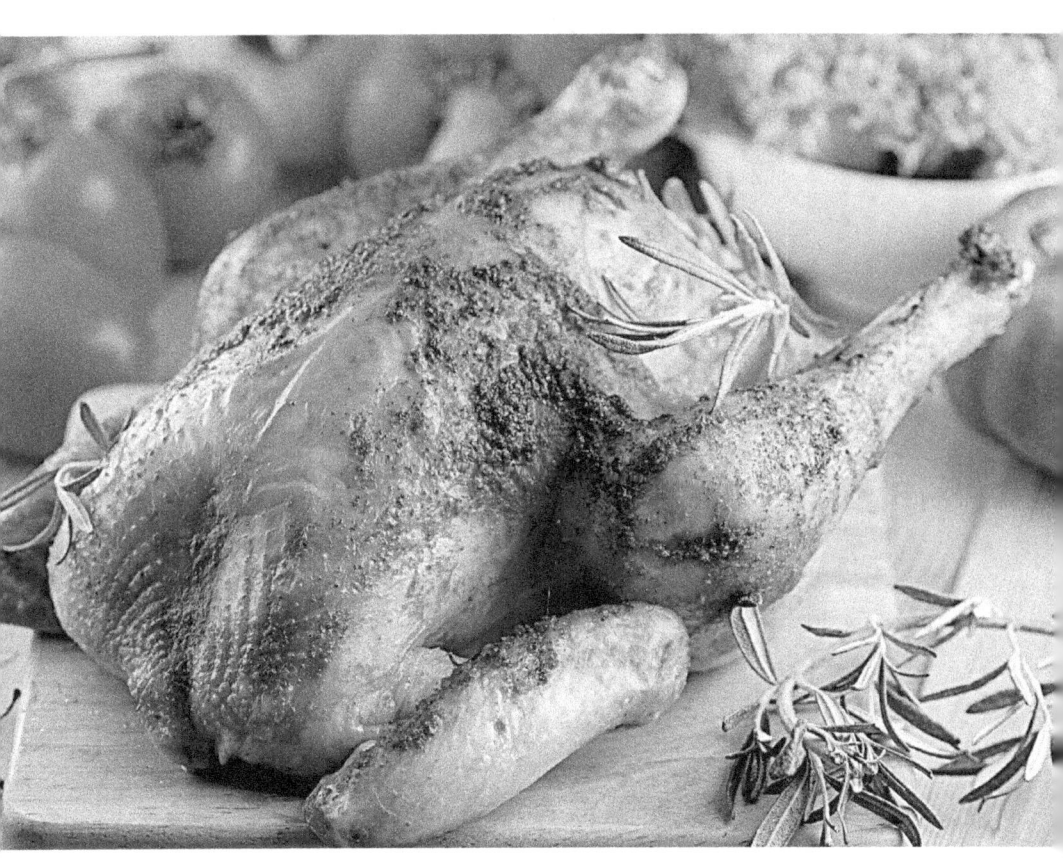

# Fig Vinegar Chicken

## Ingredients:

1. 1 garlic clove
2. 1 tablespoon honey
3. 1 tablespoon Dijon mustard
4. 1 tablespoon orange juice
5. 1 tablespoon extra-virgin olive oil
6. 2 tablespoons fig balsamic vinegar
7. ½ teaspoon SPG mix (divided ¼ teaspoon and ¼ teaspoon)
8. 4 eight-ounce boneless chicken breasts

## Preparation:

1. Puree garlic and put in a large bowl
2. Add honey, Dijon mustard, orange juice, olive oil, fig balsamic vinegar and ¼ teaspoon SPG mix to bowl and whisk together to make marinade
3. Add chicken breasts to marinade, cover with plastic and marinate in refrigerator 30 minutes to 2 hours
4. Take chicken out of refrigerator and put on counter 20 minutes prior to cooking
5. Pre-heat grill over a medium-high flame 15 minutes

## Cooking:

1. Remove chicken from marinade and season with remaining ¼ teaspoon SPG mix
2. Grill chicken 5 minutes
3. Flip chicken over and grill 5 minutes
4. Remove chicken from grill
5. Serve and enjoy

TIP: You can bake chicken 15 minutes at 400 degrees

Leftovers are great for Grilled Chicken Salad page 182

# Bacon and Maple Syrup Glazed Chicken

## Ingredients:

1. 1 small yellow onion
2. 1 garlic clove
3. ½ cup maple syrup
4. ½ cup chicken broth
5. ¼ cup balsamic vinegar
6. 1 tablespoon Dijon mustard
7. ½ teaspoon fresh lemon juice
8. 4 eight-ounce boneless chicken breasts
9. ½ teaspoon SPG mix
10. 4 slices bacon
11. 1 tablespoon extra-virgin olive oil

## Preparation:

1. Small dice onion and set aside
2. Puree garlic and set aside
3. Combine maple syrup, chicken broth, balsamic vinegar, Dijon mustard and lemon juice in a bowl, whisk together and set aside
4. Trim fat off chicken
5. Evenly season chicken with SPG mix and set aside

## Cooking:

1. Pre-heat a large sauté pan over a medium-high flame 1 minute
2. Cook bacon until crisp and remove from pan
3. Add olive oil to same pan
4. Add chicken and sauté 5 minutes
5. Flip chicken over, add onions and sauté 4 minutes
6. Add garlic and sauté 1 minute
7. Remove chicken from pan
8. Add maple syrup mixture and reduce by half
9. Return chicken to pan 30 seconds
10. Plate chicken topped with bacon and maple syrup glaze
11. Serve and enjoy

TIP: Makes a great meal with Sautéed Baby Spinach page 100 and Mashed Sweet Potatoes page 130

# Whole Roasted Chicken

## Ingredients:

1. 1 five-pound chicken
2. ½ yellow onion
3. 2 tablespoons packed fresh basil leaves
4. 5 garlic cloves
5. 1 lemon (1 tablespoon juice and rind)
6. 1 tablespoon extra-virgin olive oil
7. 2 teaspoons SPG mix

## Preparation:

1. Pre-heat oven to 350 degrees
2. Remove innards from chicken
3. Rinse chicken under cold water, pat dry with a paper towel and set aside
4. Cut onion in half and set aside
5. Tear basil leaves in half and set aside
6. Smash garlic cloves open, discard skins and add set cloves aside
7. Cut lemon in half
8. In a small bowl combine lemon juice with olive oil and evenly rub over chicken
9. Season inside and outside of chicken with SPG mix
10. Fill chicken's cavity with onion, basil, garlic and lemon rind
11. Put chicken in a roasting pan

**Cooking:**

1. Roast chicken in oven 75 minutes, until a meat thermometer reads 160 degrees
2. Remove chicken from oven and let rest 5 minutes
3. Carve chicken
4. Serve and enjoy

TIP: Goes great with Herb Baked Potatoes page 128

A nice variation is to substitute rosemary for basil or use 1 tablespoon of each

# Garlic Chicken Kebobs

## Ingredients:

1. 6 garlic cloves
2. 2 tablespoons fresh lemon juice
3. 4 tablespoons extra-virgin olive oil
4. 1 teaspoon SPG mix divided (½ teaspoon and ½ teaspoon)
5. 1 sweet onion
6. 1 pound button mushrooms
7. 2 green peppers
8. 2 red peppers
9. 2 pounds boneless chicken breasts
10. 12 skewers

## Preparation:

1. Puree garlic and put in a large mixing bowl
2. Add lemon juice, olive oil and ½ teaspoon SPG mix to bowl
3. Whisk marinade together and set aside
4. Cut onion into 1 inch squares and add to marinade
5. Trim stems off mushrooms and add caps to marinade
6. Cut peppers into 1 inch squares and add to marinade
7. Cut chicken into 1 inch squares and add to marinade
8. Mix everything together, cover bowl with plastic and marinate in refrigerator 30-60 minutes
9. If using wood skewers soak in water 30 minutes to avoid burning on grill
10. Take marinade out of refrigerator

11. Alternately skewer red pepper, onion, chicken, green pepper and mushroom twice on each skewer and set aside
12. Pre-heat grill over a medium-high flame 15 minutes
13. Evenly season kebobs with remaining ½ teaspoon SPG mix

**Cooking:**
1. Grill kebobs 4 minutes
2. Turn kebobs and grill 3 minutes
3. Turn kebobs again and grill 2 minutes
4. Remove kebobs from grill
5. Serve and enjoy

# Chicken Vesuvio

## Ingredients:

1. 1 four-pound chicken (whole or cut into eight pieces)
2. 4 garlic cloves
3. 1 pound frozen green peas
4. ½ cup white wine
5. 1 tablespoon dried oregano
6. 1 teaspoon fresh lemon juice
7. ½ teaspoon garlic powder
8. 1½ teaspoons SPG mix
9. 3 Idaho potatoes
10. ¼ cup extra-virgin olive oil

## Preparation:

1. Pre-heat oven to 400 degrees
2. Puree garlic and set aside
3. Put peas in strainer, rinse under warm water to thaw and set aside
4. Combine wine, oregano and lemon juice in a small bowl and set aside
5. Combine garlic powder and SPG mix in a small bowl and set aside
6. Cut potatoes lengthwise into 8 wedges each and set aside
7. Cut chicken into eight pieces; 2 legs, 2 thighs, 2 wings and 2 breasts
8. Evenly season potatoes and chicken with combined garlic powder and SPG mix
9. Take out a large baking sheet and set it aside

**Cooking:**

1.  Pre-heat a large sauté pan over a medium-high flame 1 minute
2.  Add olive oil and heat 30 seconds
3.  Brown both sides of chicken pieces in two batches and put on baking sheet
4.  In same pan brown all potato wedges 8-12 at a time and add to baking sheet
5.  Turn off flame and add garlic, white wine, oregano and lemon juice
6.  Evenly pour this mixture over chicken and potatoes and bake 30 minutes
7.  Set sauté pan aside to cool
8.  Once sauté pan has completely cooled add peas to absorb flavors from pan
9.  After chicken and potatoes have baked 30 minutes, add peas and bake 5 minutes
10. Remove from oven and let rest 5 minutes
11. Serve and enjoy

# Chicken Fajitas

## Ingredients:

1. 1 yellow onion
2. 1 red pepper
3. 1 green pepper
4. 2 jalapeño peppers
5. 2 garlic cloves
6. 2 pounds boneless chicken breast
7. 2 tablespoons extra-virgin olive oil
8. 2 tablespoons Mexican spice mix
9. 1 tablespoon fresh lime juice

## Preparation:

1. Thinly slice onion, red and green peppers and put in a bowl
2. Fine dice jalapeños and add to bowl
3. Puree garlic and set aside
4. Trim fat off chicken
5. Cut each chicken breast in half lengthwise
6. Slice chicken into ¼ inch wide strips and set aside

**Cooking:**

1. Pre-heat a large sauté pan over a medium-high flame 1 minute
2. Add olive oil
3. Add onions and peppers and sauté 5 minutes
4. Add garlic, chicken and Mexican spice mix and sauté 5 minutes
5. Add lime juice
6. Serve and enjoy

Fajitas are best with warmed brown rice tortillas and Guacamole page 149

# Chicken Tacos

## Ingredients:

1. 1 large red onion
2. 1 red pepper
3. 1 green pepper
4. 2 jalapeño peppers
5. 2 garlic cloves
6. 2 heaping tablespoons Mexican spice mix
7. 1½ cups tomato juice
8. ½ cup of packed fresh cilantro
9. 4 eight-ounce boneless chicken breasts
10. 2 tablespoons extra-virgin olive oil
11. 1 tablespoon fresh lime juice

## Preparation:

1. Small dice onion and put in a bowl
2. Small dice red and green peppers and add to bowl
3. Fine dice jalapeños and add to bowl
4. Puree garlic and set aside
5. Fine chop cilantro and set aside
6. Trim fat off chicken and cut each breast into two equal size pieces
7. Put chicken in a pot filled with enough water to cover by 1 inch

**Cooking:**

1. Bring pot to a boil over a high flame
2. When it reaches a boil, lower flame and simmer 5 minutes, until chicken is fully cooked
3. Strain and briefly rinse chicken
4. Shred chicken and set aside
5. Pre-heat a large sauté pan over a medium-high flame 1 minute
6. Add olive oil
7. Add onions and peppers and sauté 3 minutes
8. Add garlic and Mexican spice mix and sauté 1 minute
9. Add tomato juice, cilantro, lime juice and shredded chicken
10. Bring to a boil and simmer 3 minutes
11. Serve and enjoy

I like best with warmed soft shell corn tortillas and Guacamole page 149

# Hunter Chicken

## Ingredients:

1. ½ yellow onion
2. 8 ounces button mushrooms
3. 2 garlic cloves
4. 3 plum tomatoes
5. 4 eight-ounce chicken breasts
6. ½ teaspoon SPG mix (divided ¼ teaspoon and ¼ teaspoon)
7. 1 tablespoon packed fresh tarragon leaves
8. 2 tablespoons extra-virgin olive oil
9. 1 teaspoon fresh lemon juice
10. ½ cup chicken broth

## Preparation:

1. Small dice onion and set aside
2. Quarter mushrooms and set aside
3. Puree garlic and set aside
4. Large dice tomato and set aside
5. Trim fat off chicken
6. Evenly season chicken with ¼ teaspoon SPG mix and set aside
7. Measure tarragon and have ready to chop just prior to its use

## Cooking:

1. Pre-heat a large sauté pan over a medium-high flame 1 minute
2. Add olive oil
3. Add chicken and sauté 5 minutes
4. Add onions and mushrooms and sauté 2 minutes
5. Flip chicken over and sauté 4 minutes
6. Add garlic, tomatoes and remaining ¼ teaspoon SPG mix and sauté 1 minute
7. Fine chop tarragon
8. Add tarragon, lemon juice and chicken broth and bring to a boil
9. Serve and enjoy

TIP: You can substitute basil for tarragon and crimini mushrooms for button

# Chicken Stir Fry

## Ingredients:

1. 1 red pepper
2. 2 carrots
3. 4 ounces button mushrooms
4. 1 broccoli crown
5. 2 garlic cloves
6. 2 teaspoons ginger
7. 3 green onions
8. 2 tablespoons packed fresh basil
9. 1½ pounds boneless chicken breast
10. 1 tablespoon cornstarch
11. 1 tablespoon water
12. 2 tablespoons extra-virgin olive oil
13. 1 teaspoon SPG mix
14. ½ cup chicken broth
15. ½ cup water

## Preparation:

1. Cut pepper into ½ inch squares and put in a bowl
2. Peel carrots and cut them in half
3. Cut thicker half in half lengthwise
4. Slice carrots into ⅛ inch thick discs and add to bowl
5. Quarter mushrooms and add to bowl
6. Cut broccoli into bite-size florets and set aside separately
7. Puree garlic and put in a small bowl
8. Grate ginger and add to bowl
9. Chop white and light green parts of green onions and add to bowl
10. Chop remaining dark green onions and put in a separate bowl
11. Thinly slice basil and add to dark green onions

12. Cut chicken breasts in half lengthwise
13. Slice chicken into ¼ inch thick strips and set aside
14. Combine cornstarch and water, whisk together and set aside

## Cooking:

1. Bring two inches of water to a boil in a sauce pan
2. Add broccoli, blanch 1 minute, strain and set aside
3. Pre-heat a large sauté pan over a high flame 1 minute
4. Add olive oil and heat 20 seconds
5. Add peppers, carrots and mushrooms and sauté 3 minutes
6. Add garlic, ginger, green onion, chicken, broccoli and SPG mix and sauté 3 minutes
7. Add chicken broth and water and bring to a boil
8. Whisk cornstarch and water into stir fry
9. Bring to a boil and simmer 1 minute to thicken
10. Add remaining green onions and basil
11. Serve and enjoy

Goes great with Stir Fry Rice page 156

# Honey Mustard Chicken

## Ingredients:

1. 4 eight-ounce boneless chicken breasts
2. ¾ cup honey mustard barbeque sauce (page 52 divided ¼ cup and ½ cup)
3. ½ teaspoon SPG mix

## Preparation:

1. Put chicken and ¼ cup honey mustard barbeque sauce in a resealable plastic bag
2. Seal bag and leave on counter to marinate while grill pre-heats
3. Pre-heat grill over a medium-high flame 15 minutes
4. Remove chicken from bag and evenly season each breast with SPG mix

## Cooking:

1. Grill chicken 5 minutes
2. Rotate chicken 90 degrees, baste using remaining sauce and grill 2 minutes
3. Flip chicken over, baste with sauce and grill 5 minutes
4. Remove chicken from grill
5. Serve and enjoy

TIP: Use leftovers for Grilled Chicken Salad page 182

# Honey Mustard Barbeque Sauce

## Ingredients:

1. ½ teaspoon SPG mix
2. ½ teaspoon garlic powder
3. 1 cup honey
4. ⅔ cup yellow mustard
5. ⅓ cup distilled white vinegar

## Preparation:

1. Combine all ingredients in a saucepan and whisk together

## Cooking:

1. Bring to a boil over a medium-high flame
2. When sauce reaches a boil, lower flame and simmer 10 minutes
3. Turn off flame and let sauce cool
4. Pour sauce into a mason jar or any container with a tight lid
5. Store in refrigerator up to 1 month
6. Serve and enjoy

TIP: Try with Chicken Fingers page 54

# Chicken Fingers

## Ingredients:

1. 1 cup brown rice flour
2. 1½ teaspoons SPG mix
3. ¾ teaspoon garlic powder
4. ½ teaspoon paprika
5. ½ teaspoon dry mustard
6. ¼ teaspoon cayenne pepper
7. ¼ teaspoon freshly ground black pepper
8. 1 cup rice drink
9. 2 eight-ounce boneless chicken breasts
10. ½ cup canola oil

## Preparation:

1. Combine flour, SPG mix, garlic powder, paprika, dry mustard, cayenne pepper and black pepper in a shallow bowl, mix and set aside
2. Pour rice drink into a shallow bowl and set aside
3. Trim fat off chicken
4. Cut chicken in half lengthwise
5. Slice chicken into ¼ inch thick strips and set aside
6. Using your left hand, dip a piece of chicken into rice milk, let it drain briefly, then lay it in flour mixture
7. Using your right hand, coat chicken with flour mixture and set aside
8. Repeat steps 6 and 7 with each piece of chicken

## Cooking:

1. Pre-heat a large sauté pan over a medium-high flame 1 minute
2. Add canola oil and heat 1 minute
3. Fry chicken 2 minutes per side
4. Serve and enjoy

# Fried Chicken

## Ingredients:

1. 1 cup brown rice flour
2. 1½ teaspoons SPG mix
3. ¾ teaspoon garlic powder
4. ½ teaspoon paprika
5. ½ teaspoon dry mustard
6. ¼ teaspoon cayenne pepper
7. ¼ teaspoon freshly ground black pepper
8. 1 cup rice drink
9. 6 chicken legs
10. 6 chicken thighs
11. 1 cup canola oil

## Preparation:

1. Pre-heat oven to 350 degrees
2. Put a baking rack on a baking sheet and set aside
3. Combine flour, SPG mix, garlic powder, paprika, dry mustard, cayenne pepper and black pepper in a shallow bowl, mix and set aside
4. Pour rice drink into a shallow bowl and set aside
5. Using your fingers and a knife when needed, remove skin from chicken
6. Using your left hand, dip a piece of chicken into rice milk, let it drain briefly, then lay it in flour mixture
7. Using your right hand, coat chicken with flour mixture and set aside
8. Repeat steps 6 and 7 with each piece of chicken

**Cooking:**

1. Pre-heat a large sauté pan over a medium-high flame 1 minute
2. Add canola oil and heat 1 minute
3. Brown chicken 3-4 minutes per side and place on baking rack
4. Bake chicken 20 minutes, until a meat thermometer reads 160 degrees
5. Remove chicken from oven and let rest 5 minutes
6. Serve and enjoy

# Chapter 4 | **Pork**

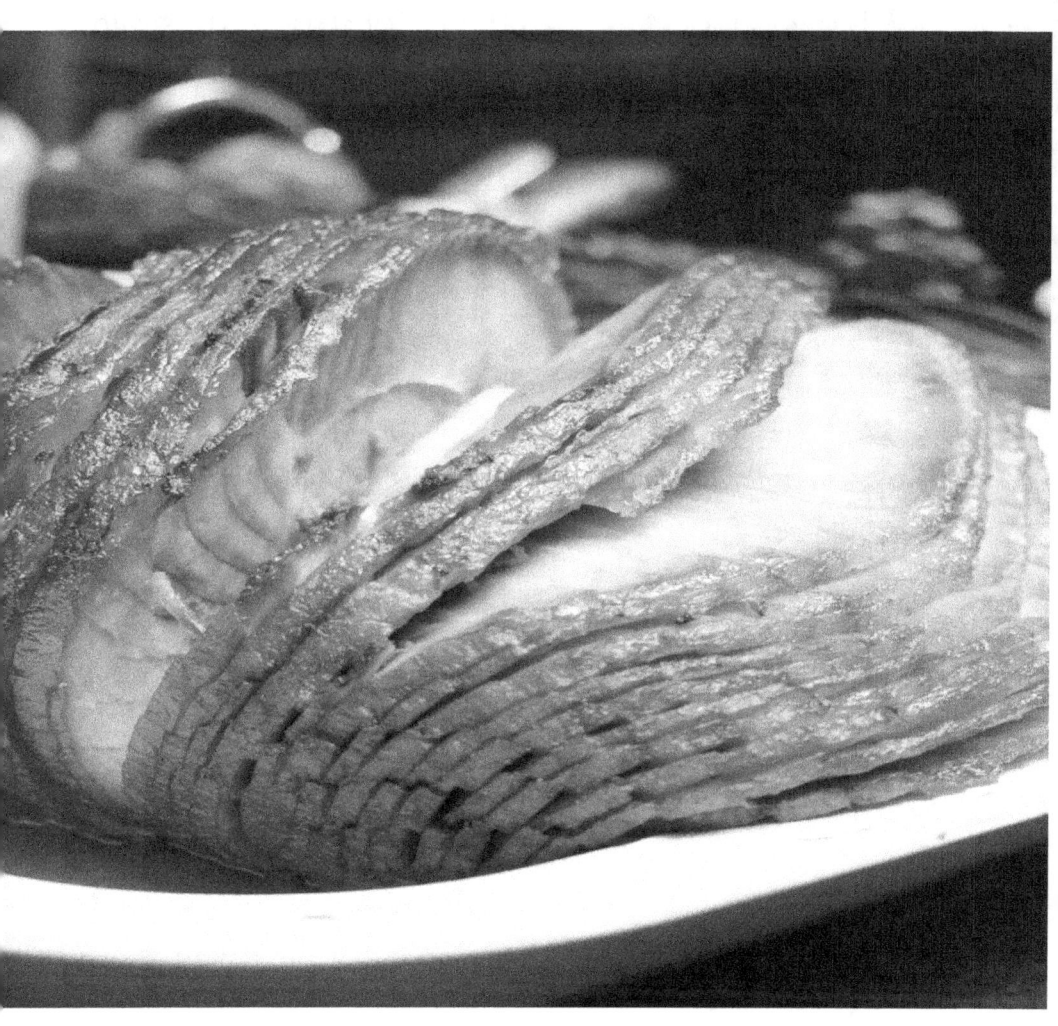

# Glazed Ham

## Ingredients:

1. 1 seven-pound smoked ham butt
2. 30 whole cloves
3. 1 cup packed light brown sugar
4. ¼ cup pineapple juice
5. 2 tablespoons stone ground mustard
6. 1 tablespoon balsamic vinegar

## Preparation:

1. Pre-heat oven to 350 degrees
2. Place ham face down on a cutting board and score sides with both vertical and horizontal cuts
3. Stud cloves in ham where score marks cross and place ham face down on a baking sheet
4. Combine sugar, juice, mustard and vinegar in a small saucepan and put on stove

## Cooking:

1. Put ham in oven
2. Whisk glaze over a medium flame until combined, about 1 minute
3. Turn flame off and set glaze aside for basting
4. After ham has baked 1 hour, baste with ½ of glaze and bake 20 minutes
5. Baste ham with remaining glaze and bake another 20 minutes
6. Remove ham from oven
7. Reserve glaze for dipping
8. Take cloves out of ham
9. Place ham face down on cutting board
10. Thinly slice ham and top with reserved glaze if desired
11. Serve and enjoy

# Rosemary Garlic Pork Chops

## Ingredients:

1. 4 eight-ounce center cut pork chops
2. 1 tablespoon packed fresh rosemary leaves, no stems
3. 2 garlic cloves
4. 2 tablespoons extra-virgin olive oil
5. 1 teaspoon SPG mix

## Preparation:

1. Take pork chops out of refrigerator and set aside
2. Fine dice rosemary and put in a bowl
3. Puree garlic and add to bowl
4. Add olive oil and SPG mix to bowl and mix to form a paste
5. Rub paste onto pork chops and set aside while grill pre-heats
6. Pre-heat grill over a medium-high flame 15 minutes

## Cooking:

1. Grill pork chops 5 minutes
2. Rotate pork chops 90 degrees and grill 2 minutes
3. Flip pork chops over and grill 5 minutes
4. Take pork chops off grill, cover with aluminum foil and let rest 5 minutes
5. Serve and enjoy

TIP:  Pork chops can be broiled on high 5 minutes on each side

# Pulled Pork

## Ingredients:

1. 1 seven-pound pork butt
2. 1 tablespoon SPG mix
3. 1 tablespoon Mexican spice mix
4. 1 tablespoon Canola oil
5. 1 cup water
6. 1 cup tomato juice
7. 3 cups barbeque sauce (divided ½ cup and 2½ cups)

## Preparation:

1. Pre-heat oven to 350 degrees
2. Combine SPG mix and Mexican spice mix
3. Evenly rub spices over pork (not on fat side)

**Cooking:**

1. Pre-heat Dutch oven over a high flame 1 minute
2. Add canola oil
3. Add pork fat side down and sear 3 minutes without touching
4. Sear remaining sides 1 minute each
5. Make sure fat side is up and add water and tomato juice
6. Pour ½ cup barbeque sauce over pork
7. Cover with lid and braise in oven 3 hours (until fork tender)
8. Remove pork from oven and let rest 10 minutes
9. Pour off any juices
10. Place pork on cutting board, discard bone and any large pieces of fat
11. Shred using 2 forks, one to hold pork still and another to pull shreds of pork away
12. Return pulled pork to Dutch oven, add remaining 2½ cups barbeque sauce, stir and bring to a boil
13. Serve and enjoy

TIP: Try pork without using remaining 2½ cups barbeque sauce and serve on warmed corn tortillas with sliced avocado and Black Bean and Corn Salad page 196

# Fried Pork Chops

## Ingredients:

1. 1 cup brown rice flour
2. 1½ teaspoons SPG mix
3. ¾ teaspoon garlic powder
4. ½ teaspoon paprika
5. ½ teaspoon dry mustard
6. ¼ teaspoon cayenne pepper
7. ¼ teaspoon freshly ground black pepper
8. ½ cup rice drink
9. 5 eight-ounce center cut pork chops
10. ½ cup canola oil

## Preparation:

1. Pre-heat oven to 350 degrees
2. Combine flour, SPG mix, garlic powder, paprika, dry mustard, cayenne pepper and black pepper in a shallow bowl, mix and set aside
3. Pour rice drink into a separate shallow bowl and set aside
4. Trim fat off pork
5. Using your left hand, dip a piece of pork into rice drink, let it drain briefly, then lay it in flour mixture
6. Using your right hand, coat pork with flour mixture and set aside
7. Repeat steps 5 and 6 with each piece of pork
8. Take out a baking sheet and set aside

## Cooking:

1. Pre-heat a large sauté pan over a medium-high flame 1 minute
2. Add canola oil and heat 1 minute
3. Brown pork chops 2-3 minutes per side and place on baking sheet
4. Bake pork chops 15 minutes, until a meat thermometer reads 160 degrees
5. Serve and enjoy

# Grilled Pork Tenderloin

## Ingredients:

1. 4 garlic cloves
2. 1 tablespoon fresh ginger
3. 3 tablespoons extra-virgin olive oil
4. 1 tablespoon fresh lime juice
5. 1 teaspoon Dijon mustard
6. 1 teaspoon SPG mix (divided ½ teaspoon and ½ teaspoon)
7. 2 1¼-pound pork tenderloins

## Preparation:

1. Puree garlic and put in a mixing bowl
2. Grate ginger and add to bowl
3. Add olive oil, lime juice, Dijon mustard and ½ teaspoon SPG mix to bowl
4. Whisk together and set marinade aside
5. Trim fat off tenderloins
6. Put tenderloins in a large resealable bag, add marinade and seal
7. Marinate in refrigerator 30 minutes to 4 hours
8. Take tenderloins out of refrigerator and set on counter
9. Pre-heat grill over a medium-high flame 15 minutes

**Cooking:**

1. Remove tenderloins from marinade and season with remaining ½ teaspoon SPG mix
2. Grill tenderloins 5 minutes
3. Turn tenderloins and grill 5 minutes
4. Turn tenderloins again and grill 5 minutes
5. Grill tenderloins 15 minutes for medium-rare and 20 minutes for medium-well
6. Remove tenderloins from grill, cover with aluminum foil and let rest 5 minutes
7. Thinly slice tenderloins
8. Serve and enjoy

TIP:  Tenderloins can be baked 20 minutes at 400 degrees

# Fig Vinegar Marinated Pork Kebobs

## Ingredients:

1. 2 garlic cloves
2. 4 tablespoons fig balsamic vinegar
3. 2 tablespoons honey
4. 2 tablespoons Dijon mustard
5. 2 tablespoons orange juice
6. 2 tablespoons extra-virgin olive oil
7. 1 teaspoon SPG mix divided (½ teaspoon and ½ teaspoon)
8. 1 yellow onion
9. 8 ounces button mushrooms
10. 2 red peppers
11. 2 pounds pork tenderloin
12. 12 skewers

## Preparation:

1. Puree garlic and put in a large mixing bowl
2. Add fig vinegar, honey, Dijon mustard, orange juice, olive oil and ½ teaspoon SPG mix to bowl and whisk together to make marinade
3. Cut onion into 1 inch squares and add to marinade
4. Trim stem off mushrooms and add caps to marinade
5. Cut peppers into 1 inch squares and add to marinade
6. Trim fat off pork
7. Cut pork into 1 inch squares and add to marinade
8. Mix everything together, cover bowl with plastic and marinate in refrigerator 30 minutes to 4 hours stirring one time halt way through

9.  If using wood skewers
    soak in water
    30 minutes to avoid
    burning on grill
10. Take marinade out of
    refrigerator
11. Alternately skewer
    onion, pork, pepper
    and mushroom twice
    on each skewer
12. Pre-heat grill over a
    medium-high flame
    15 minutes
13. Evenly season kebobs
    with remaining
    ½ teaspoon SPG mix

## Cooking:

1.  Grill kebobs 4 minutes
2.  Turn kebobs and grill 3 minutes
3.  Turn kebobs again and grill 2 minutes
4.  Remove kebobs from grill
5.  Serve and enjoy

TIP: Shish kebobs can be broiled on high 4 minutes on each side

# Roasted Center Cut Pork Loin

## Ingredients:

1. 1½ teaspoons caraway seed
2. 1½ teaspoons SPG mix
3. 1 tablespoon extra-virgin olive oil
4. 1 four-pound center cut pork loin

## Preparation:

1. Pre-heat oven to 350 degrees
2. Combine caraway seeds and SPG mix
3. Drizzle olive oil over pork and evenly season with spice mixture
4. Place pork in a roasting pan

## Cooking:

1. Roast pork in oven 2 hours, until a meat thermometer reads 160 degrees
2. Remove pork from oven, cover with aluminum foil and let rest 10 minutes
3. Slice pork
4. Serve and enjoy

TIP: Pork loin takes approximately 30 minutes per pound to cook

Goes great with Sautéed Sweet Potatoes page 134

# Chapter 5 | **Pastas**

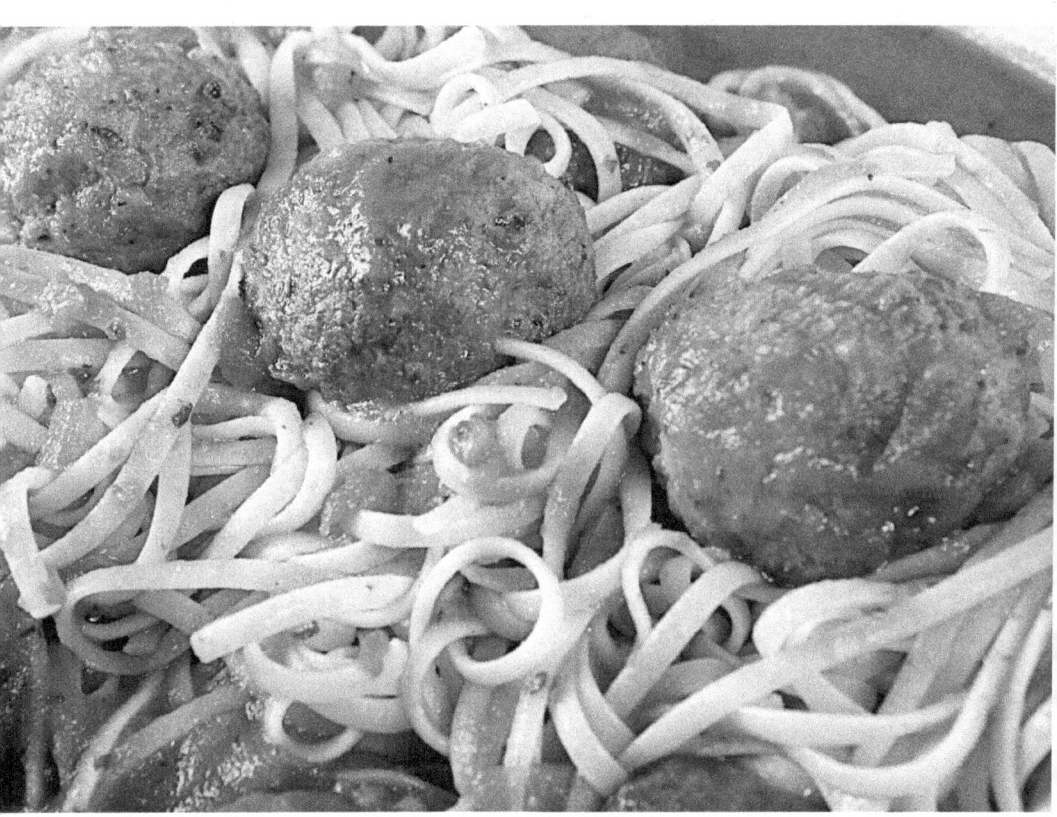

# Meat Sauce

## Ingredients:

1. 1 yellow onion
2. 1 red pepper
3. 1 green pepper
4. 3 garlic cloves
5. 1 can (28 ounces) whole peeled tomatoes
6. 1 can (28 ounces) tomato puree
7. 2 tablespoons tomato paste
8. 3 teaspoons dried basil
9. 1½ teaspoon dried oregano
10. 3 bay leaves
11. 1 pound ground beef
12. 2 teaspoons SPG mix

## Preparation:

1. Small dice onion and put in a bowl
2. Small dice peppers and add to bowl
3. Puree garlic and set aside
4. Pour tomatoes into a separate bowl and smash tomatoes into bite sized pieces with your fingers
5. Add tomato puree, tomato paste, basil, oregano and bay leaves to tomatoes and set aside

## Cooking:

1. Pre-heat a large sauté pan over a medium-high flame 1 minute
2. Add beef and sauté 4 minutes
3. Add onion and peppers and sauté 2 minutes
4. Add garlic and SPG mix and sauté 1 minute
5. Add tomato mixture and stir to combine
6. Bring to a boil, lower flame and simmer 30 minutes
7. Remove bay leaves
8. Serve and enjoy

TIP: Serve with your favorite pasta

# Marinara Sauce

## Ingredients:

1. 1 yellow onion
2. 1 red pepper
3. 1 green pepper
4. 3 garlic cloves
5. 1 can (28 ounces) whole peeled tomatoes
6. 1 can (28 ounces) tomato puree
7. 2 tablespoons tomato paste
8. 2 teaspoons dried basil
9. 1 teaspoon dried oregano
10. 3 bay leaves
11. 2 tablespoons extra-virgin olive oil
12. 1¼ teaspoons SPG mix

## Preparation:

1. Small dice onion and put in a bowl
2. Small dice peppers and add to bowl
3. Puree garlic and set aside
4. Pour tomatoes into a separate bowl and smash into bite sized pieces with your fingers
5. Add tomato puree, tomato paste, basil, oregano and bay leaves to tomatoes and set aside

## Cooking:

1. Pre-heat a large sauté pan over a medium-high flame 1 minute
2. Add olive oil
3. Add onion and peppers and sauté 4 minutes
4. Add garlic and SPG mix and sauté 1 minute
5. Add tomato mixture and stir to combine
6. Bring to a boil, lower flame and simmer 30 minutes
7. Remove bay leaves
8. Serve and enjoy

TIP: Use this sauce with Spaghetti and Meatballs page 80

# Spaghetti and Meatballs

## Ingredients:

1. 10 ounces brown rice spaghetti noodles
2. 1 pound ground beef
3. ¼ cup yellow onion
4. 1 tablespoon packed fresh flat leaf parsley
5. ¾ teaspoon SPG mix
6. ¼ teaspoon garlic powder
7. 2 tablespoons ketchup
8. 4 cups marinara sauce (page 78 or store bought)
9. 3 tablespoons extra-virgin olive oil

## Preparation:

1. Cover a large pot of water and bring to a rolling boil
2. Put ground beef in a large mixing bowl
3. Fine dice onion and add to bowl
4. Fine chop parsley and add to bowl
5. Add SPG mix, garlic powder and ketchup to bowl
6. Mix everything together using your hands
7. Roll 1 inch round meatballs and set aside

**Cooking:**

1. In a small pan, heat marinara over a medium flame
2. Add spaghetti to boiling water and cook until al dente
3. Strain spaghetti, briefly rinse and set aside
4. Pre-heat a large sauté pan over a medium-high flame 1 minute
5. Add olive oil and heat 30 seconds
6. Brown meatballs 1 minute per side
7. Add marinara and simmer 10 minutes
8. Add spaghetti and warm 2 minutes
9. Serve and enjoy

TIP:  Roll meatballs in palm of your hands not in your fingers, if the meat sticks get your hands a little wet.  Rolling 1 inch balls helps to keep them from falling apart.

# Italian Sausage and Vegetable Pasta

## Ingredients:

1. 1 sweet onion
2. 1 red pepper
3. 1 green pepper
4. 8 ounces button mushrooms
5. 2 garlic cloves
6. 1 pound bulk Italian sausage
7. 1 teaspoon SPG mix
8. ½ teaspoon dried oregano
9. ½ teaspoon dried basil
10. ¼ teaspoon dried French thyme
11. 8 ounces brown rice fusilli pasta (I prefer Tinkyada brand)
12. 3 cups marinara sauce (page 78 or store bought)
13. 1 tablespoon extra-virgin olive oil

## Preparation:

1. Cover a large pot of water and bring to a rolling boil
2. Medium dice onion and put in a bowl
3. Cut peppers into ½ inch squares and add to bowl
4. Cut mushrooms in half and add to bowl
5. Puree garlic and set aside
6. Form sausage into bite sized pieces and set aside
7. Combine SPG mix, oregano, basil and thyme in a small bowl and set aside

## Cooking:

1. Add pasta to boiling water and cook until al dente
2. Strain pasta, briefly rinse and set aside
3. In a small pan, heat marinara sauce over a medium flame
4. Pre-heat a large sauté pan over a medium-high flame 1 minute
5. Add olive oil
6. Add sausage and sauté 4 minutes
7. Add onions, peppers and mushrooms, stir and sauté 6 minutes
8. Add garlic and combined seasonings, stir and sauté 3 minutes
9. Add pasta and sauce and heat 2 minutes
10. Serve and enjoy

# Chicken, Basil and Sun-Dried Tomato Pasta

## Ingredients:

1. 1 yellow onion
2. 3 garlic cloves
3. 1 yellow squash
4. 1 green zucchini
5. 3 eight-ounce boneless chicken breasts
6. 1½ teaspoons fresh lemon zest
7. 2 tablespoons packed fresh basil leaves
8. 8 ounces brown rice pasta shells
9. 2 tablespoons extra-virgin olive oil
10. ¼ cup sun-dried tomatoes, julienne cut
11. 1 teaspoon SPG mix
12. ½ cup reserved pasta water

## Preparation:

1. Cover a large pot of water and bring to a rolling boil
2. Medium dice onion and set aside
3. Puree garlic and set aside
4. Cut ends off squash and zucchini and slice in half lengthwise
5. Lay squash and zucchini flat and slice into ¼ inch thick discs and set aside
6. Trim fat off chicken and cut each breast in half lengthwise
7. Cut chicken into ¼ inch wide strips
8. Zest lemon and put zest in a small bowl
9. Chop basil and add to bowl

**Cooking:**

1. Add pasta to boiling water and cook until al dente
2. Reserve ½ cup pasta water for later use
3. Strain pasta, briefly rinse and set aside
4. Pre-heat a large sauté pan over a medium-high flame 1 minute
5. Add olive oil
6. Add onion and sauté 3 minutes
7. Add chicken and sauté 3 minutes
8. Add garlic, squash and zucchini and sauté 2 minutes
9. Add lemon zest, basil, sun-dried tomatoes and SPG mix, stir and sauté 2 minutes
10. Add cooked pasta and reserved pasta water and bring to a boil
11. Serve and enjoy

# Herb Coated Chicken and Pasta

## Ingredients:

1. 1 cup brown rice flour
2. 1½ teaspoons SPG mix
3. ¾ teaspoon garlic powder
4. ½ teaspoon dried basil
5. ½ teaspoon dried oregano
6. ¼ teaspoon freshly ground black pepper
7. 1 cup rice drink
8. 3 eight-ounce boneless chicken breasts
9. 20 ounces marinara sauce (page 78 or store bought)
10. 8 ounces brown rice fusilli pasta
11. ¼ cup extra-virgin olive oil

## Preparation:

1. Cover a large pot of water and bring to a rolling boil
2. Combine flour, SPG mix, garlic powder, basil, oregano and black pepper in a shallow bowl, mix and set aside
3. Pour rice drink into a separate shallow bowl and set aside
4. Cut chicken breasts into three equal size pieces each
5. Place chicken pieces between layers of plastic wrap and pound to equal thickness
6. Using your left hand, dip a piece of chicken into rice milk, let it drain briefly, then lay it in flour mixture
7. Using your right hand, coat chicken with flour mixture and set aside
8. Repeat steps 6 and 7 with each piece of chicken

## Cooking:

1. In a small pan, heat marinara sauce over a medium flame
2. Add pasta to boiling water and cook until al dente
3. Strain pasta, briefly rinse and set aside
4. Pre-heat a large sauté pan over a medium-high flame 2 minutes
5. Add olive oil and heat 30 seconds
6. Add chicken and sauté 4 minutes
7. Flip chicken over and sauté 3 minutes
8. Remove chicken from pan and let rest 3 minutes
9. Add pasta to sauce and warm 2 minutes
10. Plate pasta and sauce, then top with chicken
11. Serve and enjoy

TIP: Goes great with Sautéed Red Pepper and Yellow Squash page 94

# Chapter 6 | **Vegetables**

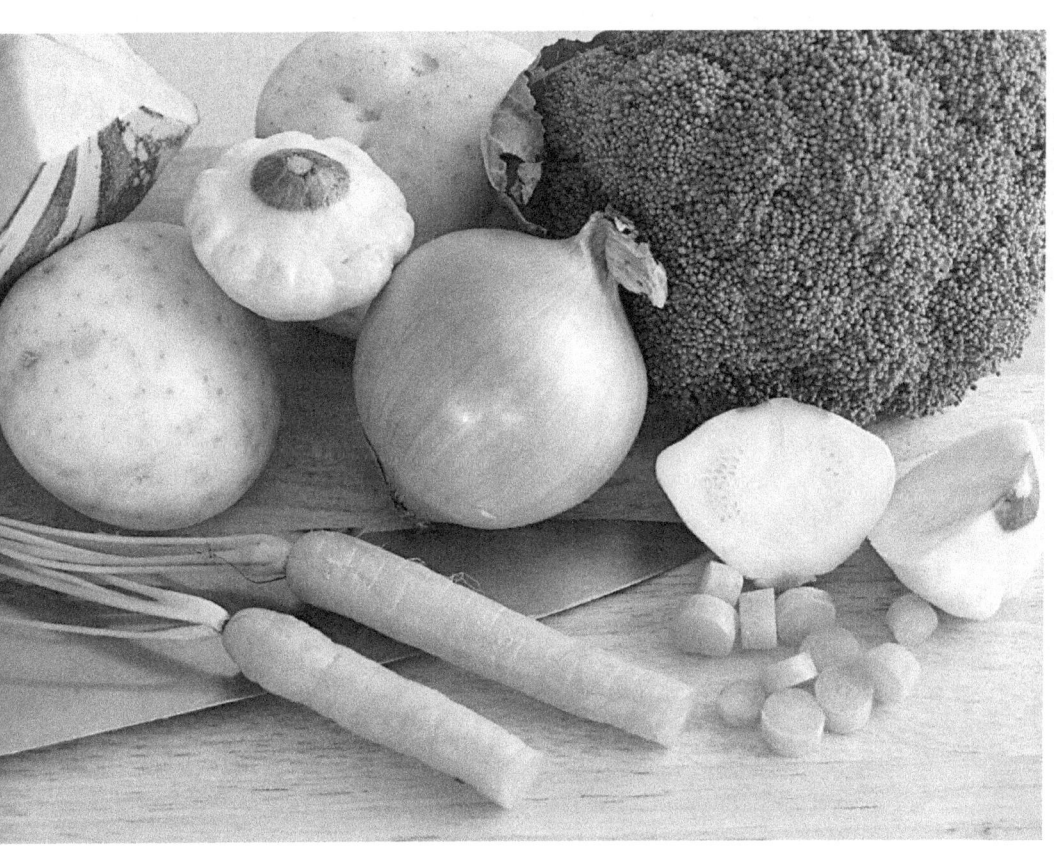

# Bacon and Balsamic Glazed Green Beans

## Ingredients:

1. 4 slices bacon
2. 1 pound green beans
3. 1 small garlic clove
4. ¼ cup yellow onion
5. ½ teaspoon SPG mix
6. 2 tablespoons packed light brown sugar
7. 1 tablespoon balsamic vinegar

## Preparation:

1. Freeze bacon 10 minutes (this makes cutting very easy)
2. Trim ends off green beans and set green beans aside
3. Puree garlic and set aside
4. Small dice onion and set aside
5. Take bacon out of freezer, slice into ¼ inch thick strips and set aside

## Cooking:

1. In a large sauté pan, bring ½ inch of water to a boil
2. Add green beans and blanch 1 minute
3. Strain green beans and set aside
4. Pre-heat same pan over a medium-high flame 1 minute
5. Add bacon and sauté 4 minutes, stirring occasionally
6. Add onions and sauté 1 minute
7. Add green beans, garlic and SPG mix and sauté 1 minute
8. Add brown sugar and vinegar, toss and sauté 1 minute
9. Serve and enjoy

# Honey Glazed Carrots

## Ingredients:

1. 1 pound carrots
2. 1 tablespoon extra-virgin olive oil
3. ¼ teaspoon SPG mix
4. 1 tablespoon honey

## Preparation:

1. Peel carrots
2. Cut each carrot in half
3. Cut thicker half in half lengthwise
4. Slice carrots into ¼ inch thick discs

**Cooking:**

1. Pre-heat a sauté pan over a medium-high flame 1 minute
2. Add olive oil
3. Add carrots and sauté 3 minutes
4. Season with SPG mix, stir and sauté 2 minutes
5. Add honey, stir and sauté 30 seconds
6. Serve and enjoy

# Sautéed Red Pepper and Yellow Squash

## Ingredients:

1. 1 small sweet onion
2. 1 red pepper
3. 2 yellow squash
4. 1 garlic clove
5. 1 tablespoon extra-virgin olive oil
6. ¼ teaspoon SPG mix

## Preparation:

1. Small dice onion and put in a bowl
2. Cut red pepper into thin strips and add to onions
3. Cut ends off squash and slice in half lengthwise
4. Lay squash flat and slice into ¼ inch thick discs and set aside
5. Puree garlic and set aside

**Cooking:**

1. Pre-heat a large sauté pan over a medium-high flame 1 minute
2. Add olive oil
3. Add onions and red peppers and sauté 4 minutes
4. Add squash, garlic and SPG mix and sauté 3 minutes
5. Serve and enjoy

# Sautéed Mixed Vegetables

## Ingredients:

1. 1 pound green beans
2. 6 ounces shitake mushrooms
3. 1 red pepper
4. 2 tablespoons extra-virgin olive oil
5. ½ teaspoon SPG mix
6. ¼ teaspoon garlic powder

## Preparation:

1. Trim ends off green beans and set green beans aside
2. Pull stems completely off mushrooms
3. Slice mushrooms into thin strips and put in a bowl
4. Slice pepper into thin strips and add to bowl

## Cooking:

1. In a large sauté pan, bring ½ inch of water to a boil
2. Add green beans and blanch 1 minute
3. Strain green beans and set aside
4. Pre-heat same pan over a medium-high flame 1 minute
5. Add olive oil
6. Add mushrooms and red peppers and sauté 3 minutes
7. Add green beans, SPG mix and garlic powder and sauté 2 minutes
8. Serve and enjoy

# Corn O'Brien

## Ingredients:

1. 1 pound frozen corn kernels
2. ½ cup red pepper
3. ½ cup green pepper
4. 1 small garlic clove
5. 1 tablespoon extra-virgin olive oil
6. ½ teaspoon SPG mix

## Preparation:

1. Put corn in a strainer and run under warm water to thaw and set aside
2. Small dice peppers and set aside
3. Puree garlic and set aside

## Cooking:

1. Pre-heat a sauté pan over a medium-high flame 1 minute
2. Add olive oil
3. Add peppers and sauté 2 minutes
4. Add corn, garlic and SPG mix and sauté 3 minutes
5. Serve and enjoy

TIP:  For spicy corn substitute Mexican spice mix for SPG mix

# Sautéed Baby Spinach

## Ingredients:

1. ½ yellow onion
2. 1 garlic clove
3. 1 tablespoon extra-virgin olive oil
4. 12 ounces baby spinach
5. ½ teaspoon SPG mix
6. 1 teaspoon fresh lemon juice

## Preparation:

1. Small dice yellow onion and set aside
2. Puree garlic and set aside

**Cooking:**

1. Pre-heat a large sauté pan over a medium-high flame 1 minute
2. Add olive oil
3. Add onion and sauté 2 minutes
4. Add garlic, spinach and SPG mix and sauté 3 minutes
5. Add lemon juice, stir and sauté 1 minute
6. Serve and enjoy

# Carrots and Green Beans

## Ingredients:

1. 1 pound carrots
2. 1 pound green beans
3. 1 tablespoon extra-virgin olive oil
4. ½ teaspoon SPG mix
5. ¼ teaspoon garlic powder

## Preparation:

1. Peel carrots
2. Julienne carrots and set aside
3. Trim ends off green beans and set aside

**Cooking:**

1. Bring ½ inch water to boil in a large sauté pan
2. Add carrots and blanch 30 seconds
3. Add green beans to carrots and blanch 1 minute
4. Strain carrots and green beans
5. Pre-heat same sauté pan over a medium-high flame 1 minute
6. Add olive oil
7. Add carrots, green beans, SPG mix and garlic powder
8. Sauté 3 minutes
9. Serve and enjoy

# Sautéed Mushrooms

## Ingredients:

1. 1 small yellow onion
2. 1 pound button mushrooms (you can substitute crimini mushrooms)
3. 1 garlic clove
4. 3 tablespoons extra-virgin olive oil
5. ½ teaspoon SPG mix
6. ¼ teaspoon dried tarragon leaves

## Preparation:

1. Medium dice yellow onion and set aside
2. Tear stems off mushrooms and set mushrooms aside
3. Puree garlic and set aside

**Cooking:**

1. Pre-heat a large sauté pan over a medium flame 1 minute
2. Add olive oil
3. Add onions and sauté 3 minutes
4. Add mushrooms and sauté 3 minutes
5. Flip mushrooms over and sauté 2 minutes
6. Turn flame to low
7. Add garlic, SPG mix and tarragon and sauté 4 minutes
8. Serve and enjoy

# Steamed Broccoli

## Ingredients:

1. 1 pound broccoli crowns
2. ½ teaspoon fresh lemon juice
3. ¼ teaspoon SPG mix

## Preparation:

1. Cut broccoli into 1 inch by 1 inch florets
2. Use a 2-quart sauce pan with lid
3. Fill pan with ½ inch of water and put on stove

**Cooking:**

1. Bring water to a boil over a high flame
2. Add broccoli
3. Cover with lid and steam 3 minutes
4. Strain broccoli
5. Drizzle with lemon juice and season with SPG mix
6. Serve and enjoy

# Cauliflower

## Ingredients:

1. 1 head cauliflower
2. ½ teaspoon SPG mix

## Preparation:

1. Cut cauliflower into 2 inch by 2 inch florets
2. Fill a large pot with hot water and put on stove

## Cooking:

1. Bring water to a rolling boil over a high flame
2. Add cauliflower and cook 3 minutes
3. Strain cauliflower and season with SPG mix
4. Serve and enjoy

# Asparagus, Yellow Squash and Carrots

## Ingredients:

1. ½ pound fresh asparagus
2. 1 yellow squash
3. ½ pound carrots
4. 1 tablespoon extra-virgin olive oil
5. ½ teaspoon SPG mix

## Preparation:

1. Pre-heat oven to 400 degrees
2. Hold ends of a piece of asparagus and try to touch them together, wherever asparagus breaks is where it is tender
3. Cut remaining asparagus at this point and place on a baking sheet
4. Cut squash into ⅓ inch by ⅓ inch by 2 inch pieces and add to baking sheet
5. Peel carrots
6. Cut carrots into ¼ inch by ¼ inch by 2 inch batons, just thinner than squash and add to baking sheet
7. Evenly drizzle vegetables with olive oil and season with SPG mix

## Cooking:

1. Bake vegetables 10 minutes
2. Remove from oven
3. Serve and enjoy

TIP:  Double this recipe and make it during the holidays

# Acorn Squash

### Ingredients:

1. 2 acorn squash
2. 2 teaspoons extra-virgin olive oil
3. ½ teaspoon SPG mix

### Preparation:

1. Pre-heat oven to 400 degrees
2. Cut each squash in half
3. Scoop out seeds
4. Evenly drizzle open side of squash with olive oil and season with SPG mix
5. Place open side down on a baking sheet

**Cooking:**

1. Bake squash 50 minutes, until fork tender
2. Remove from oven
3. Cut each piece of squash in half
4. Serve and enjoy

TIP: Goes great with Glazed Ham page 60 and Bacon and Maple Syrup Glazed Chicken page 34

# Grilled Zucchini and Yellow Squash

## Ingredients:

1. 2 green zucchini
2. 2 yellow squash
3. 2 tablespoons extra-virgin olive oil
4. ½ teaspoon SPG mix
5. 2 tablespoons packed fresh basil
6. ½ teaspoon fresh lemon juice

## Preparation:

1. Cut ends off zucchini and squash
2. Cut ¼ inch thick slices on a long diagonal and put on a platter
3. Drizzle zucchini and squash with olive oil and season with SPG mix
4. Thinly slice basil and set aside
5. Pre-heat grill over a medium-high flame 15 minutes

**Cooking:**

1. Grill zucchini and squash 3 minutes on each side
2. Remove from grill
3. Top with basil and lemon juice
4. Serve and enjoy

# Baby Broccoli

## Ingredients:

1. 1 pound baby broccoli
2. 1 teaspoon extra-virgin olive oil
3. ¼ teaspoon SPG mix

## Preparation:

1. Trim ¼ inch off all broccoli stems
2. Pre-heat grill over a medium-high flame 15 minutes

## Cooking:

1. In a large sauté pan bring ½ inch of water to a boil over a high flame
2. Add broccoli and blanch 1 minute
3. Strain broccoli, pat dry and put on a plate
4. Drizzle broccoli with olive oil and season with SPG mix
5. Grill 3 minutes on each side
6. Serve and enjoy

TIP: I love the char flavor from the grill with this, but you can also cook baby broccoli in boiling water 3 minutes, then strain and season with SPG mix

# Corn on the Cob

## Ingredients:

1. 5 ears of corn
2. 1 tablespoon extra-virgin olive oil
3. ½ teaspoon SPG mix

## Preparation:

1. Completely husk corn
2. Drizzle corn with olive oil and season with SPG mix

## Cooking:

1. Pre-heat grill over a medium flame 15 minutes
2. Grill corn 3 minutes on each side (9-12 minutes)
3. When corn is slightly charred and tender remove from grill
4. Serve and enjoy

TIP: You can pierce a kernel of corn with a fork to check tenderness

# Spicy Corn on the Cob

## Ingredients:

1. 5 ears of corn
2. 1 tablespoon Mexican spice mix
3. 1 tablespoon extra-virgin olive oil

## Preparation:

1. Completely husk corn
2. Combine Mexican spice mix and olive oil in a small bowl and form a paste
3. Evenly rub paste over each ear of corn

## Cooking:

1. Pre-heat grill over a medium-high flame 15 minutes
2. Cook corn 3 minutes on each side (9-12 minutes)
3. When corn is slightly charred and tender remove from grill
4. Serve and enjoy

TIP: You can pierce a kernel of corn with a fork to check tenderness

# Grilled Portabella Mushrooms

## Ingredients:

1. 4 portabella mushrooms
2. 2 tablespoons extra-virgin olive oil
3. ½ teaspoon SPG mix

## Preparation:

1. Tear stem off each mushroom
2. Scrape gills off each mushroom with a spoon and place mushrooms on a platter
3. Drizzle olive oil on both sides of mushrooms and season with SPG mix

**Cooking:**

1. Pre-heat grill over a medium-high flame 15 minutes
2. Grill mushrooms 3 minutes
3. Flip mushrooms over and grill 3 minutes
4. Serve and enjoy

TIP:  You can also bake 15 minutes at 400 degrees

# Grilled Asparagus

## Ingredients:

1. 1 pound fresh asparagus
2. ½ tablespoon extra-virgin olive oil
3. ½ teaspoon SPG mix
4. ½ teaspoon fresh lemon juice

## Preparation:

1. Hold ends of a piece of asparagus and try to touch them together, wherever asparagus breaks is where it is tender
2. Cut remaining asparagus at this point and put on a platter
3. Drizzle asparagus with olive oil
4. Season with SPG mix
5. Pre-heat grill over a medium-high flame 15 minutes

## Cooking:

1. Grill asparagus 3 minutes on each side
2. Remove asparagus from grill and drizzle with lemon juice
3. Serve and enjoy

TIP: Asparagus can also be broiled in oven on high 3-4 minutes

# Chapter 7 | **Sides**

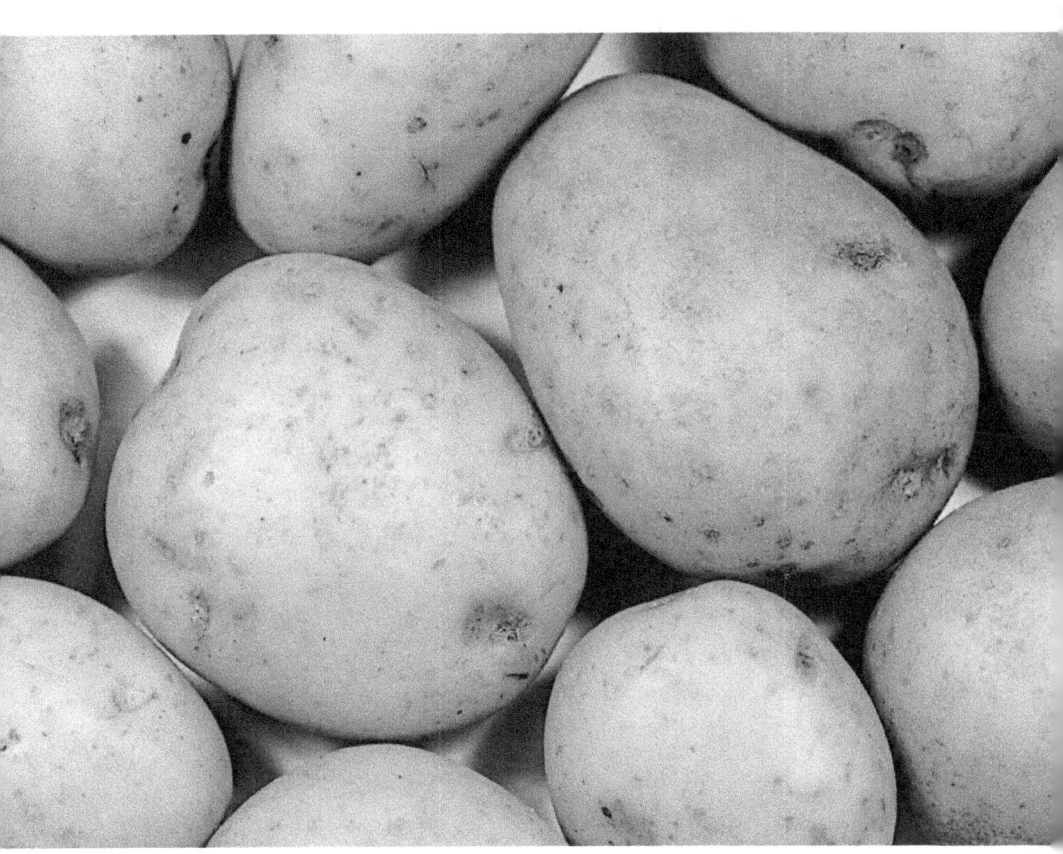

# Herb Baked Potatoes

## Ingredients:

1. 2 Idaho potatoes
2. 1 teaspoon SPG mix
3. ½ teaspoon dried oregano
4. ½ teaspoon dried basil
5. ¼ teaspoon dried French thyme
6. ¼ teaspoon garlic powder
7. 2 tablespoons canola oil

## Preparation:

1. Pre-heat oven to 400 degrees
2. Wash and dry potatoes
3. Combine SPG mix, oregano, basil, thyme and garlic powder in a small bowl and set aside
4. Pour canola oil on a non-stick baking sheet
5. Dice potatoes into ¼ by ½ inch pieces
6. Evenly season potatoes with spice mixture
7. Arrange potatoes in a single layer on baking sheet

**Cooking:**

1. Bake potatoes 45 minutes
2. Serve and enjoy

# Mashed Sweet Potatoes

### Ingredients:

1. 2 large sweet potatoes
2. 1½ tablespoons packed light brown sugar
3. ½ teaspoon SPG mix

### Preparation:

1. Pre-heat oven to 400 degrees
2. Tightly wrap potatoes with aluminum foil

## Cooking:

1. Place potatoes seal side up on a baking sheet
2. Bake potatoes 60-75 minutes, until they easily dent when squeezed
3. Remove foil and scrape skin off potatoes with fork
4. Put sweet potato in a shallow bowl
5. Add brown sugar and SPG mix and completely mash potatoes with your fork
6. Serve and enjoy

TIP: Ideal with Glazed Ham page 60 or Bacon and Maple Syrup Glazed Chicken page 34

# Mashed Yukon Gold Potatoes

## Ingredients:

1. 3 pounds Yukon gold potatoes
2. 3 green onions
3. 1½ teaspoons SPG mix
4. ½ teaspoon garlic powder
5. ⅔ cup extra-virgin olive oil

## Preparation:

1. Peel potatoes
2. Cut any larger potatoes in half
3. Put potatoes in a large pot and fill with water
4. Chop green onions and set aside

## Cooking:

1. Bring pot to a boil over a high flame
2. When it reaches a boil, turn flame to low and simmer 15 minutes (until potatoes are fork tender)
3. Strain potatoes and return to pot
4. Over a medium-high flame cook moisture out of potatoes 1 minute
5. Mash potatoes (I believe using a ricer makes the best mashed potatoes)
6. Add green onions, SPG mix, garlic powder and olive oil to potatoes and combine
7. Serve and enjoy

# Sautéed Sweet Potato

## Ingredients:

1. 2 sweet potatoes
2. 2 tablespoons extra-virgin olive oil
3. ½ teaspoon SPG mix
4. 2 teaspoons light brown sugar

## Preparation:

1. Dice sweet potatoes into ¼ inch squares

**Cooking:**

1. Pre-heat a large sauté pan over a medium-high flame 1 minute
2. Add olive oil
3. Add sweet potatoes and sauté 2 minutes
4. Stir potatoes and turn flame down to medium and sauté 5 minutes
5. Season with SPG mix and stir potatoes
6. Continue to cook 5-10 minutes stirring occasionally until potatoes are fork tender
7. Evenly sprinkle brown sugar over potatoes and stir until sugar is dissolved
8. Serve and enjoy

TIP: If sugar does not fully dissolve, add a little more olive oil and stir

# Rosemary Potato Wedges

## Ingredients:

1. 3 Idaho potatoes
2. 1 tablespoon packed fresh rosemary leaves, no stems
3. 2 garlic cloves
4. 1 teaspoon SPG mix
5. 1 teaspoon fresh lemon zest
6. 3 tablespoons extra-virgin olive oil

## Preparation:

1. Pre-heat oven to 350 degrees
2. Wash and dry potatoes
3. Cut each potato lengthwise into 8 wedges
4. Fine chop rosemary and set aside
5. Puree garlic and set aside
6. Zest lemon and set aside
7. Take out a baking sheet

**Cooking:**

1. Pre-heat a large sauté pan over a medium-high flame 1 minute
2. Add olive oil and heat 30 seconds
3. Add 12 potato wedges and brown each side (about 2 minutes per side)
4. Remove potatoes to baking sheet and brown remaining potatoes
5. Once browned, return all potatoes to pan
6. Add rosemary, garlic, SPG mix and lemon zest
7. Gently toss potatoes and spread on baking sheet
8. Bake potatoes 25 minutes
9. Serve and enjoy

# Rustic Spiced Potatoes

## Ingredients:

1. 1 red pepper
2. 1 carrot
3. 2 pounds baby red potatoes
4. 4 tablespoons extra-virgin olive oil
5. 1 teaspoon SPG mix
6. ½ teaspoon garlic powder
7. ¼ teaspoon Mexican spice mix

## Preparation:

1. Small dice red pepper and put in a bowl
2. Peel carrot
3. Small dice carrot and add to bowl
4. Medium dice potatoes

## Cooking:

1. Pre-heat a large sauté pan over a medium-high flame 1 minute
2. Add olive oil
3. Add potatoes and sauté 10 minutes, stirring occasionally
4. Add peppers and carrots and sauté 10 minutes, stirring occasionally
5. Add SPG mix, garlic powder and Mexican spice mix and sauté 5 minutes
6. Serve and enjoy

# Parsley Potatoes

## Ingredients:

1. 2 pounds baby red potatoes
2. 1 tablespoon packed fresh Italian parsley
3. ½ teaspoon SPG mix
4. ¼ teaspoon garlic powder
5. 1 tablespoon extra-virgin olive oil

## Preparation:

1. Medium dice potatoes
2. Put potatoes in a large pot and fill with water
3. Chop parsley and set aside

**Cooking:**

1. Bring pot to a boil over a high flame
2. When it reaches a boil, lower flame and simmer 15 minutes
3. Strain potatoes and return to same pot
4. Over a medium-high flame cook moisture out of potatoes 1 minute
5. Add parsley, SPG mix, garlic powder and olive oil
6. Gently stir and heat 2 minutes
7. Serve and enjoy

# Potatoes with Bacon and Onion

## Ingredients:

1. 5 slices bacon
2. 1 yellow onion
3. 2 Idaho potatoes
4. 2 tablespoons extra-virgin olive oil
5. ½ teaspoon SPG mix
6. ½ teaspoon garlic powder
7. ¼ teaspoon freshly ground black pepper

## Preparation:

1. Freeze bacon 10 minutes
2. Medium dice onion and set aside
3. Dice potatoes into ¼ by ½ inch pieces
4. Take bacon out of freezer, slice into ¼ inch thick strips and set aside

## Cooking:

1. Pre-heat a large sauté pan over a medium-high flame 1 minute
2. Add olive oil and heat 30 seconds
3. Add potatoes and sauté 10 minutes stirring occasionally
4. Add onion and bacon and sauté 10 minutes stirring occasionally
5. Add SPG mix, garlic powder and black pepper and sauté 5 minutes
6. Serve and enjoy

# Shoestring French Fries

## Ingredients:

1. 2 Idaho potatoes
2. approximately 32 ounces corn oil
3. 1 teaspoon SPG mix

## Preparation:

1. Fill Dutch oven one inch high with corn oil
2. Heat oil to 375 degrees over a high flame
3. Pre-heat oven to 250 degrees
4. Lay a wire cooling rack on a baking sheet
5. Have a large slotted spoon ready to strain fries out of oil
6. Use a mandolin or knife to slice potatoes into $\frac{1}{8}$ by $\frac{1}{8}$ by 3 inch strips

## Cooking:

1. Never add more than 1 cup of fries at a time to avoid oil overflow
2. When oil's temperature is 375 degrees add 1 cup of fries and back away
3. Fry 4 minutes, until fries are crispy and bubbling has subsided
4. Strain onto prepared baking sheet and season with SPG mix
5. Return oil's temperature to 375 degrees and repeat steps 1, 2, 3 and 4
6. You can keep fries warm in a 250 degree oven while you continue cooking more
7. Serve and enjoy

TIP: You want to fry at 350 degrees, but when you add potatoes, oil temperature will drop. If it drops too low, potatoes will absorb oil and become soggy instead of frying in it, and becoming crispy

# Sweet Potato Fries

## Ingredients:

1. 2 sweet potatoes
2. approximately 32 ounces corn oil
3. 1 teaspoon SPG mix

## Preparation:

1. Lay a wire cooling rack on a baking sheet
2. Have a large slotted spoon ready to strain fries out of oil
3. Fill Dutch oven one inch high with corn oil
4. Pre-heat oil to 375 degrees over a high flame
5. Use a mandolin or knife to slice potatoes into $\frac{1}{8}$ by $\frac{1}{8}$ by 3 inch thick strips

## Cooking:

1. Never add more than 1 cup of fries at a time to avoid overflow
2. When oil's temperature is 375 degrees add 1 cup of fries and back away
3. Fry 2 minutes, until fries are crispy and bubbling has subsided
4. Strain onto prepared baking sheet and season with SPG mix
5. Return oil's temperature to 375 degrees and repeat steps 1, 2, 3 and 4
6. Serve and enjoy

TIP: You want to fry at 350 degrees, but when you add potatoes, oil temperature will drop. If it drops too low potatoes will absorb oil and become soggy instead of frying in it, and becoming crispy

# Pico de Gallo

## Ingredients:

1. 4 plum tomatoes
2. ⅓ cup red onion
3. 1 jalapeño pepper
4. ½ garlic clove
5. 2 tablespoons packed fresh cilantro
6. 1 teaspoon fresh lime juice
7. ½ teaspoon SPG mix

## Preparation:

1. Medium dice tomatoes and put in a mixing bowl
2. Fine dice onion and add to bowl
3. Fine dice jalapeño and add to bowl
4. Puree garlic and add to bowl
5. Chop cilantro and add to bowl
6. Add lime juice and SPG mix to bowl
7. Mix ingredients together
8. Serve and enjoy

# Guacamole

## Ingredients:

1. 2 plum tomatoes
2. 1 tablespoon red onion
3. 1 jalapeño pepper
4. ½ garlic clove
5. 1 tablespoon packed fresh cilantro
6. ½ tablespoon fresh lime juice
7. ½ teaspoon SPG mix
8. 2 Haas avocados

## Preparation:

1. Medium dice tomatoes and put in a mixing bowl
2. Fine dice onion and add to bowl
3. Fine dice jalapeño and add to bowl
4. Puree garlic and add to bowl
5. Fine chop cilantro and add to bowl
6. Add lime juice and season with SPG mix
7. In a separate bowl mash avocados with a fork
8. Combine tomato mixture with mashed avocados
9. Serve and enjoy

# Refried Beans

## Ingredients:

1. ½ cup yellow onion
2. 1 jalapeño pepper
3. 1 garlic clove
4. 1 can (16 ounces) refried beans
5. 1 tablespoon extra-virgin olive oil
6. 1 teaspoon Mexican spice mix

## Preparation:

1. Small dice onion and set aside
2. Small dice jalapeño and set aside
3. Puree garlic and set aside
4. Open refried beans and set aside

**Cooking:**

1. Pre-heat a sauté pan over a medium-high flame 1 minute.
2. Add olive oil
3. Add onion and sauté 3 minutes
4. Add jalapeño, garlic and Mexican spice mix and sauté 1 minute
5. Add refried beans
6. Stir ingredients together and sauté 2 minutes
7. Serve and enjoy

# Spanish Rice

## Ingredients:

1. ½ cup yellow onion
2. 2 carrots
3. 1 garlic clove
4. ½ cup frozen green peas
5. 2 tablespoons packed fresh cilantro
6. 1 tablespoon extra-virgin olive oil
7. 1 cup long grain white rice
8. 1 tablespoon Mexican spice mix
9. 1 cup water
10. 1 cup tomato juice

## Preparation:

1. Small dice onion and put in a bowl
2. Peel carrots
3. Small dice carrots and add to bowl
4. Puree garlic and set aside
5. Thaw peas and set aside
6. Chop cilantro and set aside

**Cooking:**

1. Pre-heat a 2-quart pan over a medium-high flame 1 minute
2. Add olive oil
3. Add onions and carrots and sauté 2 minutes
4. Add garlic and sauté 1 minute
5. Add rice and Mexican spice mix and sauté 20 seconds
6. Add water and tomato juice
7. Stir and bring to a boil
8. When it reaches a boil, lower flame, cover with a tight fitting lid and simmer 15 minutes
9. Remove pan from flame and stir in peas and cilantro
10. Cover and let stand 5 minutes
11. Fluff rice with a fork
12. Serve and enjoy

# Saffron Rice

## Ingredients:

1. ⅓ cup yellow onion
2. 2 tablespoons extra-virgin olive oil
3. ½ teaspoon saffron threads
4. ½ teaspoon SPG mix
5. ½ teaspoon garlic powder
6. 1 cup long grain white rice
7. 2 cups chicken broth

## Preparation:

1. Small dice onion and set aside

**Cooking:**

1. Pre-heat a 2-quart pan over a medium-high flame 1 minute
2. Add olive oil
3. Add onion and sauté 2 minutes
4. Add saffron, SPG mix and garlic powder and sauté 1 minute
5. Add rice and broth
6. Stir and bring to a boil
7. When it reaches a boil, lower flame, cover with a tight fitting lid and simmer 15 minutes
8. Remove pan from flame and let rice stand, covered 5 minutes
9. Fluff rice with a fork
10. Serve and enjoy

# Stir Fry Rice

## Ingredients:

1. 1 tablespoon extra-virgin olive oil
2. 1 tablespoon sugar
3. 1 tablespoon rice wine vinegar
4. 1 cup long grain white rice
5. 2 cups water
6. ½ teaspoon SPG mix

## Cooking:

1. Combine all ingredients in a 2-quart pan
2. Bring to a boil over a high flame
3. When it reaches a boil, lower flame, cover with a tight fitting lid and simmer 15 minutes
4. Remove pan from flame and let rice stand, covered 5 minutes
5. Fluff rice with a fork
6. Serve and enjoy

# Basil Ginger Rice

## Ingredients:

1. ¼ cup yellow onion
2. 1 teaspoon fresh ginger
3. 1 garlic clove
4. 2 tablespoons packed fresh basil
5. 1 tablespoon extra-virgin olive oil
6. ½ teaspoon SPG mix
7. 1 cup long grain white rice
8. 2 cups water
9. 1 tablespoon sugar
10. 1 tablespoon rice wine vinegar

## Preparation:

1. Small dice onion and set aside
2. Grate ginger and set aside
3. Puree garlic and set aside
4. Measure basil (do not slice until needed)

## Cooking:

1. Pre-heat a 2-quart pan over a medium-high flame 1 minute
2. Add olive oil
3. Add onions and sauté 3 minutes
4. Add ginger and garlic, stir and sauté 1 minute
5. Add SPG mix, rice, water, sugar and vinegar and bring to a boil
6. When it reaches a boil, lower flame, cover with a tight fitting lid and simmer 15 minutes
7. Remove pan from flame
8. Thinly slice basil and stir into rice
9. Cover and let rice stand 5 minutes
10. Fluff rice with a fork
11. Serve and enjoy

# Chapter 8 | **Soups**

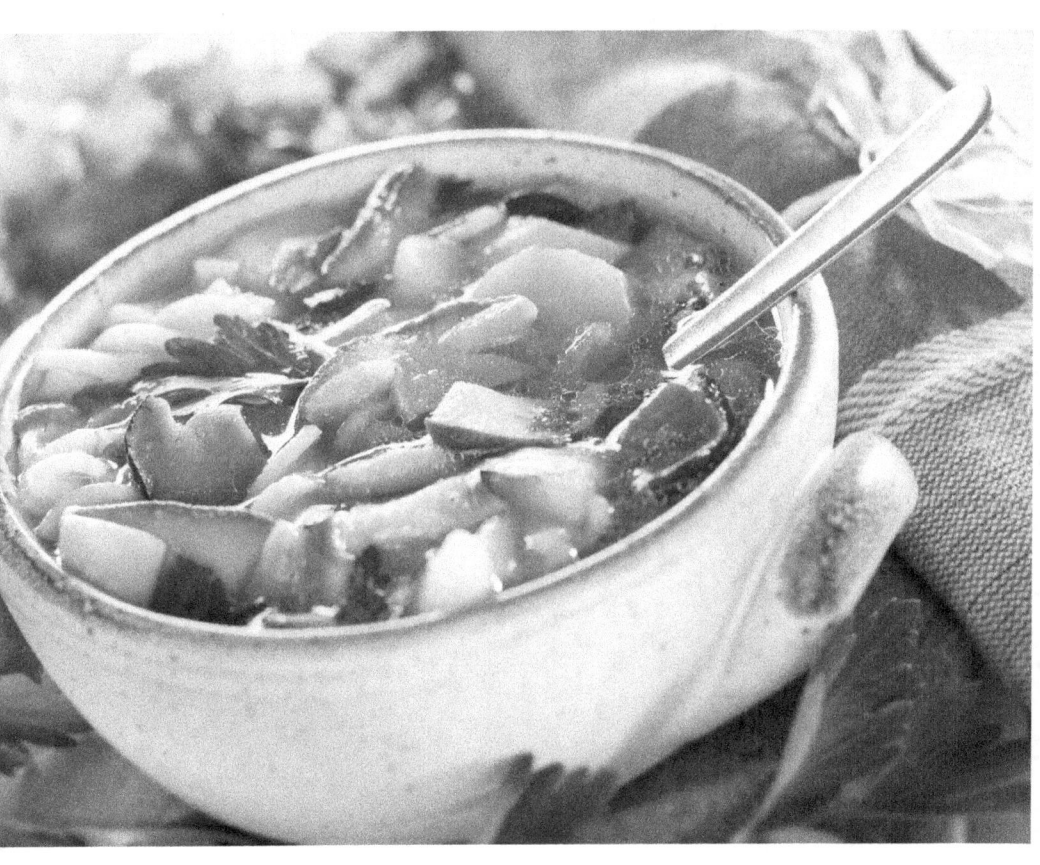

# Mushroom Soup

## Ingredients:

1. 1 yellow onion
2. 1½ pounds button mushrooms
3. 1 teaspoon SPG mix
4. 1 teaspoon dried tarragon
5. ½ teaspoon dried French thyme
6. ½ teaspoon freshly ground black pepper
7. ½ teaspoon garlic powder
8. 3 bay leaves
9. 3 tablespoons extra-virgin olive oil
10. 6 cups chicken broth

## Preparation:

1. Small dice onion and put in a bowl
2. Slice mushrooms and set aside
3. Combine SPG mix, tarragon, thyme, black pepper, garlic powder and bay leaves in a small bowl and set aside

**Cooking:**

1. Pre-heat a pot over a medium-high flame 1 minute
2. Add olive oil
3. Add onions and sauté 3 minutes
4. Add mushrooms and sauté 3 minutes
5. Add seasonings, stir and sauté 1 minute
6. Add chicken broth and bring to a boil
7. When it reaches a boil, lower flame and simmer 15 minutes
8. Remove all bay leaves
9. Serve and enjoy

# Chicken Tortilla Soup

## Ingredients:

1. 12 six-inch corn tortillas
2. 1 yellow onion
3. 1 red pepper
4. 1 green pepper
5. 2 jalapeño peppers
6. 3 garlic cloves
7. ½ cup packed fresh cilantro
8. 2 eight-ounce boneless chicken breasts
9. 2 tablespoons canola oil
10. 1 tablespoon Mexican spice mix
11. 3 cans (14.5 ounces each) whole peeled tomatoes
12. 8 cups chicken broth
13. ½ teaspoon SPG mix
14. 1 large avocado

## Prepration:

1. Pre-heat oven to 400 degrees
2. Cut 6 tortillas into 1 inch squares and set aside
3. Cut 6 tortillas into ⅛ inch thick by 2 inch long strips and place on a baking sheet
4. Small dice onion and put in a bowl
5. Small dice peppers and add to bowl
6. Puree garlic and add to bowl
7. Dice cilantro and set aside
8. Trim fat off chicken and cut each breast into two equal size pieces
9. Put chicken in a pot filled with enough water to cover by 1 inch and set on stove

## Cooking:

1. Bring pot to a boil over a high flame
2. When it reaches a boil, lower flame and simmer 5 minutes, until chicken is fully cooked
3. Strain and rinse chicken
4. Shred chicken and set aside
5. Pre-heat a large pot over a medium-high flame 1 minute
6. Add canola oil
7. Add tortilla squares and sauté 3 minutes
8. Add onions, peppers, garlic and Mexican spice mix and sauté 3 minutes
9. Add tomatoes, chicken broth and cilantro and bring to a boil
10. When it reaches a boil, lower flame and simmer 20 minutes
11. Bake tortilla strips in oven 10 minutes (until crisp)
12. Remove tortilla strips from oven, season with SPG mix and set aside
13. Puree soup in small batches using a countertop blender or an immersion blender
14. Dice avocado
15. Top each bowl of soup with shredded chicken, crisp tortilla strips and avocado
16. Serve and enjoy

# Three-Bean Chili

## Ingredients:

1. 2 pounds ground beef
2. 1 large yellow onion
3. 1 green pepper
4. 1 red pepper
5. 2 jalapeno peppers
6. 2 garlic cloves
7. 2 tablespoons Mexican spice mix
8. 1½ tablespoons ground cumin
9. 1½ tablespoons chili powder
10. 1 can (15 ounces) pinto beans
11. 1 can (15 ounces) kidney beans
12. 1 can (15 ounces) black beans
13. 1 can (15 ounces) diced tomatoes
14. 2 tablespoons tomato paste
15. 1½ cups tomato juice

## Preparation:

1. Small dice onion and put in a bowl
2. Small dice red and green peppers and add to bowl
3. Fine dice jalapeño peppers and add to bowl
4. Puree garlic and add to bowl
5. Add Mexican spice mix, cumin and chili powder to bowl and set aside
6. Strain each can of beans and set aside

**Cooking:**

1. Pre-heat a large pot over a medium-high flame 1 minute
2. Add ground beef and cook 5 minutes
3. Add onion, peppers, garlic and spices and cook 5 minutes
4. Add beans, tomatoes, tomato paste and tomato juice and bring to a boil
5. When it reaches a boil, lower flame and simmer 30 minutes
6. Serve and enjoy

# Beef Stew

## Ingredients:

1. 2 yellow onions
2. 2 Idaho potatoes
3. ¾ pound carrots
4. 4 garlic cloves
5. 2 pounds chuck steak
6. 4 tablespoons cornstarch
7. 3 tablespoons water
8. 3 tablespoons extra-virgin olive oil
9. ¼ teaspoon SPG mix
10. ½ teaspoon dried French thyme
11. 3 dried bay leaves
12. 2 tablespoons tomato paste
13. 2 teaspoons balsamic vinegar
14. 5 cups beef broth

## Preparation:

1. Small dice onions and set aside
2. Peel and small dice potatoes
3. Put potatoes in sink or separate bowl and cover with water
4. Peel carrots
5. Dice carrots same size as potatoes and set aside
6. Puree garlic and set aside
7. Trim fat off steak and cut into ½ inch cubes
8. Combine cornstarch and water, whisk together and set aside

## Cooking:

1. Pre-heat a stock pot over a high flame 1 minute
2. Add olive oil
3. Add steak and sear 3 minutes
4. Add onions and sauté 2 minutes
5. Add garlic, SPG mix, thyme and bay leaves and sauté 2 minutes
6. Add tomato paste, balsamic vinegar and beef broth and bring to a boil
7. When it reaches a boil, lower flame and simmer 20 minutes
8. Strain potatoes
9. Add potatoes and carrots and return to a boil
10. When it reaches a boil, lower flame and simmer 15 minutes
11. Remove bay leaves
12. Whisk cornstarch and water into stew
13. Bring to a boil and simmer 5 minutes
14. Serve and enjoy

# Potato Soup

## Ingredients:

1. 2 green onions
2. 1 yellow onion
3. 3 carrots
4. 1 red pepper
5. 4 Idaho potatoes (about 3½ pounds)
6. 4 tablespoons cornstarch
7. 3 tablespoons water
8. 5 slices bacon
9. 2 tablespoons extra-virgin olive oil
10. 1 teaspoon SPG mix
11. 1 teaspoon dried French thyme
12. ½ teaspoon garlic powder
13. 3 bay leaves
14. ¼ teaspoon freshly ground black pepper
15. 6 cups chicken broth

## Preparation:

1. Chop green onions and set aside for later use
2. Small dice yellow onion and put in a bowl
3. Peel carrots
4. Small dice carrots and add to bowl
5. Small dice red pepper and add to bowl
6. Peel and small dice potatoes
7. Put potatoes in sink or a separate bowl and cover with water
8. Combine cornstarch and water, whisk together and set aside

## Cooking:

1. Cook bacon until crisp
2. Crumble bacon and set aside for later use
3. Pre-heat a large pot over a medium-high flame 1 minute
4. Add olive oil
5. Add yellow onions, carrots and red peppers and sauté 2 minutes
6. Add SPG mix, thyme, garlic powder, bay leaves and black pepper and sauté 1 minute
7. Strain potatoes
8. Add potatoes and chicken broth to pot and bring to a boil
9. When it reaches a boil, lower flame and simmer 15 minutes
10. Whisk cornstarch and water into soup
11. Bring to a boil and simmer 5 minutes
12. Remove bay leaves
13. Top each bowl of soup with crumbled bacon and chopped green onions
14. Serve and enjoy

# Black Bean Soup

## Ingredients:

1. 1 yellow onion
2. 1 red pepper
3. 1 green pepper
4. 2 jalapeño peppers
5. 2 garlic cloves
6. 2 cans (30 ounces each) black beans
7. 2 tablespoons packed fresh cilantro
8. 4 tablespoons cornstarch
9. 3 tablespoon water
10. 2 tablespoons extra-virgin olive oil
11. 2 tablespoons Mexican spice mix
12. 5 cups chicken broth
13. 3 bay leaves

## Preparation:

1. Small dice onion, red pepper and green pepper and put in a bowl
2. Fine dice jalapeños and add to bowl
3. Puree garlic and set aside
4. Strain beans and set aside
5. Chop cilantro and set aside
6. Combine cornstarch and water, whisk together and set aside

## Cooking:

1. Pre-heat a pot over a medium-high flame 1 minute
2. Add olive oil
3. Add onions and peppers and sauté 4 minutes
4. Add garlic and Mexican spice mix, stir and sauté 1 minute
5. Add beans, chicken broth, bay leaves and cilantro and bring to a boil
6. When it reaches a boil, lower flame and simmer 10 minutes
7. Whisk cornstarch and water into soup
8. Bring to a boil and simmer 3 minutes
9. Remove all bay leaves
10. Serve and enjoy

# Tomato Basil Soup

## Ingredients:

1. 1 yellow onion
2. 2 carrots
3. 1 tablespoon extra-virgin olive oil
4. 1 teaspoon SPG mix
5. 1 teaspoon dried basil
6. ½ teaspoon garlic powder
7. ¼ teaspoon dried French thyme
8. 3 bay leaves
9. 4 cups tomato juice
10. 2 cups chicken broth

## Preparation:

1. Small dice onion and put in a bowl
2. Peel carrots
3. Small dice carrots and add to bowl

## Cooking:

1. Pre-heat a pot over a medium-high flame 1 minute
2. Add olive oil
3. Add onions and carrots and sauté 3 minutes
4. Add SPG mix, basil, garlic powder, thyme and bay leaves and sauté 1 minute
5. Add tomato juice and chicken broth and bring to a boil
6. When it reaches a boil, lower flame and simmer 20 minutes
7. Remove bay leaves
8. Serve and enjoy

# French Onion Soup

## Ingredients:

1. 3 large sweet onions
2. 2 tablespoons extra-virgin olive oil
3. 1 teaspoon dried French thyme
4. ½ teaspoon garlic powder
5. ½ teaspoon SPG mix
6. 3 bay leaves
7. 1 cup red wine
8. 4 cups beef broth

## Preparation:

1. Julienne onions and set aside

**Cooking:**

1. Pre-heat stock pot over a medium-high flame 2 minutes
2. Add olive oil and heat 30 seconds
3. Add onions and sauté 3 minutes without stirring or moving pot
4. Stir onions and sauté 5 minutes
5. Add thyme, garlic powder, and SPG mix and sauté 5 minutes
6. Add bay leaves and red wine
7. Reduce wine to 2 tablespoons
8. Add beef broth and bring to a boil
9. When it reaches a boil, lower flame and simmer 20 minutes
10. Remove bay leaves
11. Serve and enjoy

# Chapter 9 | **Salads**

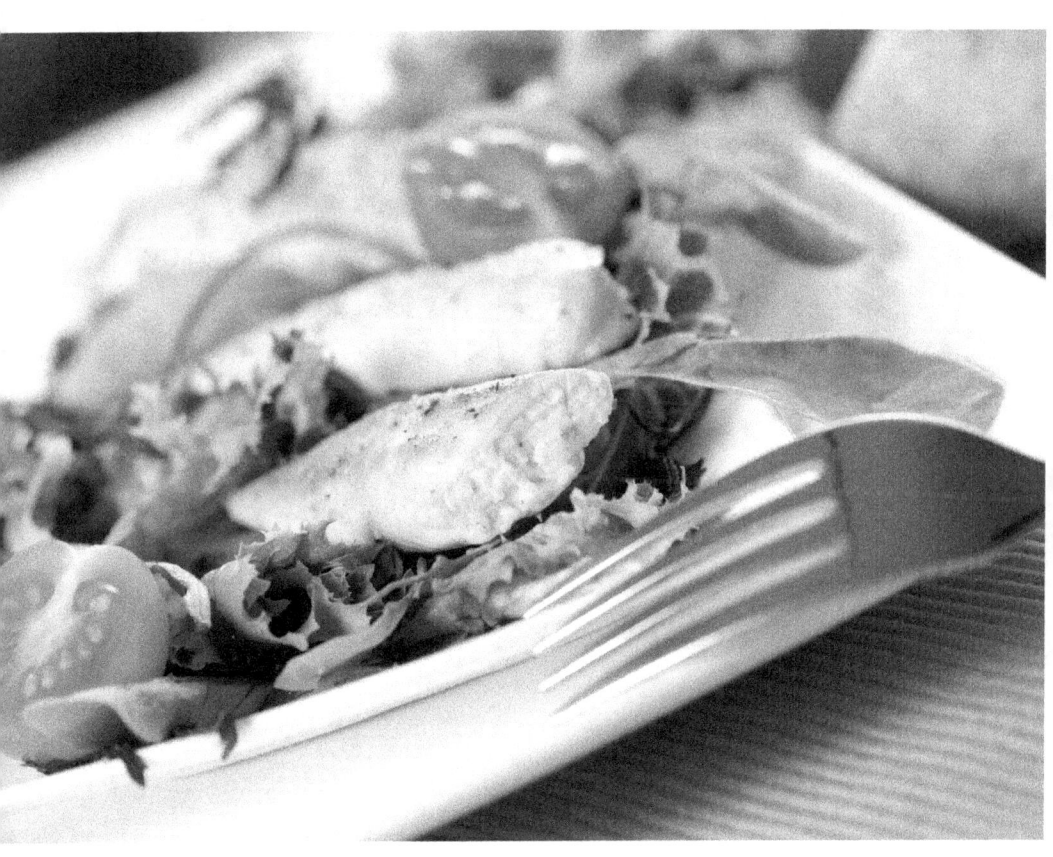

# Balsamic Vinaigrette

## Ingredients:

1. ½ garlic clove
2. ¼ cup plus
   1 tablespoon
   balsamic vinegar
3. 2 teaspoons Dijon
   mustard
4. 2 teaspoons honey
5. ½ teaspoon fresh
   lemon juice
6. ¼ teaspoon SPG mix
7. ⅛ teaspoon freshly
   ground black pepper
8. ½ cup extra-virgin
   olive oil

## Preparation:

1. Puree garlic and put in
   a mixing bowl
2. Add balsamic vinegar,
   Dijon mustard, honey,
   lemon juice, SPG mix
   and black pepper
   and whisk together
3. While whisking, slowly
   add olive oil to
   emulsify
4. Serve and enjoy

# Honey Mustard Vinaigrette

## Ingredients:

1. 5 tablespoons honey
2. 3 tablespoons Dijon mustard
3. 2 tablespoons white wine vinegar
4. ¼ teaspoon SPG mix
5. ¼ teaspoon garlic powder
6. ¼ teaspoon fresh lemon juice

## Preparation:

1. Combine all ingredients in a bowl and whisk together
2. Serve and enjoy

# Grilled Chicken Salad

## Ingredients:

1. 1 large head Romaine lettuce
2. 2 vine ripened tomatoes
3. 1 small red pepper
4. ¼ cup balsamic vinaigrette page 180
5. 2 eight-ounce boneless chicken breasts
6. 1 teaspoon SPG mix (divided ½ teaspoon and ¼ teaspoon)
7. ½ teaspoon fresh lemon juice
8. 1 avocado

## Preparation:

1. Pre-heat grill over a medium-high flame 15 minutes
2. Cut lettuce into 1 inch squares
3. Put lettuce into a large mixing bowl and refrigerate
4. Medium dice tomatoes and set aside
5. Slice red pepper into thin strips and set aside
6. Prepare vinaigrette if needed
7. Season both sides of chicken breasts with ½ teaspoon SPG mix

## Cooking:

1. Grill chicken 5 minutes
2. Flip chicken over and grill 5 minutes
3. Remove chicken from grill, drizzle with lemon juice and let rest 5 minutes
4. Remove lettuce from refrigerator
5. Medium dice avocado
6. Add avocado, tomatoes and red peppers to lettuce
7. Season salad with remaining ¼ teaspoon SPG mix
8. Cut chicken breasts in half lengthwise, slice chicken into thin strips and add to salad
9. Drizzle vinaigrette around edges of mixing bowl and toss salad
10. Serve and enjoy

TIP: Leftover Fig Vinegar Chicken page 32 and Honey Mustard Chicken page 50 are perfect for use in this salad

# Portabella Mushroom Salad

## Ingredients:

1. 1 large head Romaine lettuce
2. 16 cherry tomatoes
3. 1 small red pepper
4. 1 tablespoon packed fresh basil
5. 3 portabella mushrooms
6. 1½ tablespoons extra-virgin olive oil
7. ¾ teaspoon SPG mix (divided ½ teaspoon and ¼ teaspoon)
8. ¼ cup balsamic vinaigrette page 180

## Preparation:

1. Cut lettuce into 1 inch squares
2. Put lettuce into a large mixing bowl and refrigerate
3. Pre-heat grill over a medium-high flame 15 minutes
4. Cut tomatoes in half and set aside
5. Slice red pepper into thin strips and set aside
6. Measure basil (do not slice until needed)
7. Tear stem off each mushroom
8. Scrape gills off each mushroom with a spoon and place mushrooms on a platter
9. Drizzle mushrooms with olive oil and season with ½ teaspoon SPG mix
10. Prepare vinaigrette if needed

## Cooking:

1. Grill mushrooms 3 minutes
2. Flip mushrooms over and grill 3 minutes
3. Remove mushrooms from grill and let rest 3 minutes
4. Remove lettuce from refrigerator
5. Thinly slice basil
6. Add tomatoes, red peppers and basil to lettuce
7. Season salad with remaining ¼ teaspoon SPG mix
8. Slice mushrooms into ¼ inch squares and add to salad
9. Drizzle vinaigrette around edges of bowl and toss salad
10. Serve and enjoy

TIP: You can bake portabella mushrooms 15 minutes at 350 degrees

# Spinach and Bacon Salad with Warm Vinaigrette

## Ingredients:

1. 8 ounces baby spinach
2. 1 carrot
3. ½ teaspoon SPG mix (divided ¼ teaspoon and ¼ teaspoon)
4. ½ cup red onion
5. 8 ounces button mushrooms
6. 3 tablespoons cider vinegar
7. 2 teaspoons Dijon mustard
8. 2 teaspoons sugar
9. ¼ teaspoon freshly ground black pepper
10. 6 slices bacon
11. 2 tablespoons extra-virgin olive oil
12. canola oil if needed

## Preparation:

1. Put spinach in a large mixing bowl
2. Peel and shred carrot and add to bowl
3. Season with ¼ teaspoon SPG mix and refrigerate
4. Thinly slice onion and set aside
5. Slice mushrooms and set aside
6. In a medium bowl combine cider vinegar, Dijon mustard, sugar and black pepper
7. Whisk together and set aside

**Cooking:**

1. Cook bacon in a large sauté pan over a medium-high flame until crisp
2. Crumble bacon and set aside
3. Pour bacon grease into a measuring cup and set cup aside
4. Return pan to a medium-high flame and add olive oil
5. Add onions, mushrooms and remaining ¼ teaspoon SPG mix and sauté 4 minutes
6. If needed, add canola oil to bacon grease to equal ⅓ cup total
7. Whisk this mixture into cider vinegar mixture to make vinaigrette
8. Add vinaigrette to sauté pan and heat 30 seconds
9. Take spinach out of refrigerator
10. Pour onions, mushrooms and vinaigrette over spinach and toss
11. Top each salad with crumbled bacon
12. Serve and enjoy

# Mandarin Orange and Avocado Salad with Parsley Vinaigrette

**Ingredients:**

1. 1 head romaine lettuce
2. 2 stalks celery
3. ½ red pepper
4. 1 can (11 ounces) Mandarin oranges
5. 1 large Haas avocado
6. 1 tablespoon packed fresh Italian flat leaf parsley
7. 2 tablespoons sugar
8. ¼ cup canola oil
9. 2 tablespoons white wine vinegar
10. ½ teaspoon SPG mix

**Preparation:**

1. Cut lettuce into 1 inch squares
2. Put lettuce in a large mixing bowl and refrigerate
3. Slice celery into ⅛ inch wide pieces on a diagonal and set aside
4. Slice pepper same size as celery and set aside
5. Drain oranges and set aside
6. Medium dice avocado and set aside
7. Put parsley, sugar, canola oil, vinegar and SPG mix in a blender
8. Blend dressing on high 30 seconds
9. Remove lettuce from refrigerator and add celery, peppers, oranges and avocado
10. Pour ⅔'s of dressing around edges of bowl and toss salad

11. Plate salads and drizzle with extra dressing if desired
12. Serve and enjoy

# Garden Fresh Salad with Honey Mustard Vinaigrette

## Ingredients:

1. 1 head romaine lettuce
2. 5 slices bacon
3. ¼ cup honey mustard vinaigrette page 181
4. 2 vine ripened tomatoes
5. 2 green onions
6. 1 avocado
7. ¼ teaspoon SPG mix

## Preparation:

1. Cut lettuce into 1 inch squares
2. Put lettuce in a large mixing bowl and refrigerate
3. Cook bacon until crisp
4. Crumble bacon and set aside
5. Prepare vinaigrette if needed
6. Medium dice tomatoes and set aside
7. Chop green onions and set aside
8. Medium dice avocado and set aside
9. Remove lettuce from refrigerator
10. Add tomatoes, green onions and avocado and season with SPG mix
11. Drizzle vinaigrette around edges of bowl and toss salad

12. Top each salad with
    crumbled bacon
13. Serve and enjoy

# Hot Potato Salad

## Ingredients:

1. 3 pounds baby red potatoes
2. 4 green onions
3. ¼ cup plus 1 tablespoon cider vinegar
4. 1 tablespoon Dijon mustard
5. 1 tablespoon sugar
6. ½ teaspoon freshly ground black pepper
7. ½ pound bacon
8. canola oil if needed
9. 1 teaspoon SPG mix
10. ¼ teaspoon garlic powder

## Preparation:

1. Put potatoes in a large pot, fill with water and set on stove
2. Chop green onions and set aside
3. In a large bowl combine cider vinegar, Dijon mustard, sugar and black pepper
4. Whisk together and set aside

**Cooking:**

1. Cook bacon in a large sauté pan over a medium-high flame until crisp
2. Crumble bacon and set aside
3. Pour bacon grease into a measuring cup
4. If needed, add canola oil to bacon grease to equal ½ cup total
5. Whisk this mixture into cider vinegar mixture to make a vinaigrette and set aside
6. Bring pot of potatoes to a boil over a high flame
7. When it reaches a boil, lower flame and simmer 15 minutes
8. Strain potatoes and save pot for later use
9. Large dice potatoes
10. Return potatoes to pot they cooked in
11. Add bacon, green onions, SPG mix, garlic powder and vinaigrette and gently stir
12. Heat 2 minutes over a medium flame
13. Serve and enjoy

# Pasta Salad

**Ingredients:**

1. ½ cup balsamic vinaigrette (page 180 or store bought)
2. 1 red pepper
3. 1 green pepper
4. 1 vine ripened tomato
5. ¼ cup red onion
6. 1 tablespoon packed fresh basil
7. 1 eight-ounce boneless chicken breast
8. 8 ounces brown rice fusilli pasta
9. ½ teaspoon SPG mix

**Preparation:**

1. Cover a large pot of water and bring to a rolling boil
2. Make balsamic vinaigrette if needed
3. Cut peppers into ¼ inch squares and put in a large bowl
4. Medium dice tomato and add to bowl
5. Slice red onion as thinly as possible and add to bowl
6. Thinly slice basil, add to bowl and set aside
7. Cut chicken into two equal size pieces
8. Put chicken in a pot filled with enough water to cover by 1 inch and set on stove

## Cooking:

1. Add pasta to large pot of boiling water
2. Cook pasta until al dente
3. Strain pasta, briefly rinse and set aside to cool
4. Bring pot with chicken to a boil
5. When it reaches a boil, lower flame and simmer 5 minutes, until chicken is fully cooked
6. Strain chicken, rinse and set aside to cool
7. When chicken has cooled, cut into ¼ inch cubes and add to bowl of vegetables
8. Add cooked pasta, SPG mix and vinaigrette to bowl and toss
9. Serve and enjoy

# Black Bean and Corn Salad

## Ingredients:

1. 1 can (15 ounces) black beans
2. 1 cup frozen corn
3. ½ red pepper
4. 1 jalapeño pepper
5. 1 tablespoon packed fresh cilantro
6. 2 teaspoons balsamic vinegar
7. ½ teaspoon fresh lime juice
8. ¼ teaspoon SPG mix

## Preparation:

1. Strain and rinse beans
2. Put beans in a large mixing bowl
3. Thaw corn under running water, strain and add to bowl
4. Small dice red pepper and add to bowl
5. Fine dice jalapeño and add to bowl
6. Chop cilantro and add to bowl
7. Add balsamic vinegar, lime juice and SPG mix to bowl and toss
8. Serve and enjoy

TIP: I like to eat with Pulled Pork page 64

## COMMONLY USED TERMS:

**Al dente-** cooked foods (usually vegetables and pasta) that are prepared firm to the bite, not soft or mushy

**Batons-** foods cut into matchstick shapes of ¼ inch x ¼ inch x 2-2½ inches

**Blanch-** very briefly or partially cooking food in boiling water or hot fat

**Braise-** a combination cooking method in which foods are first browned in hot fat, then covered and slowly cooked in a small amount of liquid.

**Caramelize-** the process of cooking sugars, the browning of sugar enhances the flavor and appearance of foods

**Chiffonade-** to finely slice or shred leafy vegetables or herbs

**Dutch oven-** a heavy pot with an arched lid used for cooking pulled pork, beef brisket, etc.

**Immersion blender-** a hand held electric blender used to puree soups and sauces

**Heaping-** to fill to overflowing

**Julienne-** to cut foods into stick-shaped pieces, approximately ⅛ inch x ⅛ inch x 1-2 inches

**Mandolin-** a stainless steel, hand-operated slicing device with adjustable blades

**Puree-** Blending, mashing or straining food to achieve a smooth pulp

**Reduce-** to cook a liquid mixture, often a sauce, until its quantity decreases; typically done to concentrate flavors and thicken liquids

**Rest-** the process of using a short period of time (usually 5-20 minutes) to allow juices to settle into meat prior to carving

**Ricer-** a sieve-like utensil with small holes through which soft food is forced; it produces particles about the size of a grain of rice

**Rough chop-** to cut foods into no specific size or shape
**Sauté-** a process of cooking food in a hot pan with the aid of hot fat; cooking is usually done quickly over high temperature
**Score-** to cut shallow gashes across the surface of a food before cooking
**Sear-** to brown food quickly over high heat; usually done as a preparatory step for combination cooking methods
**Shingle-** to slightly overlap the edge of two pieces of food
**Slurry-** a mixture of raw starch and cold liquid used for thickening
**Zest-** the thin colored parts of a citrus peel

www.ingramcontent.com/pod-product-compliance
Lightning Source LLC
Chambersburg PA
CBHW060619290526
45793CB00001B/77